MIRACLE HERBS

Other Books by Dr. Stephen Holt

Soya for Health
The Soy Revolution
The Shark Cartilage Alternative for Bone and Joint Health (with M. Fuerst)
The Power of Cartilage (with J. Barilla)
Andrographis paniculata: A Monograph (with J. Barilla)
The Alcohol Clinical Index (with H.A. Skinner)

Other Books co-authored by Linda Comac

Sharks Don't Get Cancer
Sharks Still Don't Get Cancer

MIRACLE HERBS

How Herbs Combine With
Modern Medicine to
Treat Cancer, Heart Disease,
AIDS, and More

Stephen Holt, M.D.
and Linda Comac, M.A.

With a Foreword by
Thomas V. Taylor, M.D., FRCS,
Professor and Chief of General Surgery, V.A. Hospital,
Baylor College of Medicine, Houston, Texas

A BIRCH LANE PRESS BOOK
PUBLISHED BY CAROL PUBLISHING GROUP

A Birch Lane Press Book
Published by Carol Publishing Group
Birch Lane Press is a registered trademark of Carol Communications, Inc.

Editorial, sales and distribution, rights and permissions inquiries should be addressed to Carol Publishing Group, 120 Enterprise Avenue, Secaucus, N.J. 07094.

In Canada: Canadian Manda Group, One Atlantic Avenue, Suite 105, Toronto, Ontario, M6K 3E7

Carol Publishing Group books may be purchased in bulk at special discounts for sales promotion, fundraising, or educational purposes. Special editions can be created to specifications. For details, contact Special Sales Department, Carol Publishing Group, 120 Enterprise Avenue, Secaucus, N.J. 07094.

Manufactured in the United States of America
10 9 8 7 6 5 4 3 2 1

Library of Congress Cataloging-in-Publication Data

Holt, Stephen, 1950–
    Miracle herbs : how herbs combine with modern medicine to treat
cancer, heart disease, AIDS, and more / Stephen Holt and Linda Comac
: with a foreword by Thomas V. Taylor.
        p.   cm.
    Includes bibliographical references and index.
    ISBN 1–55972–463–3 (hc)
    1. Herbs — Therapeutic use.   2. Alternative medicine.   3. Cancer —
Alternative treatment.   4. Heart — Diseases — Alternative treatment.
5. AIDS (Disease) — Alternative treatment.   I. Comac, Linda.
II. Title.
RM666.H33H65   1998
615'.321 — dc21   98–4556
                                                              CIP

Contents

Foreword

Miracle Herbs, by Dr. Stephen Holt and Linda Comac, is not just another herbal book. Stephen Holt and Linda Comac have produced a groundbreaking account of the promise that herbal and botanical therapy holds for modern medicine. After thirty years as a practicing surgeon, teacher, and researcher, I have begun to recognize many of the limitations of conventional medical interventions. I continue to practice allopathic medicine, but I have become increasingly interested in the ever-increasing evidence that remedies of natural origin and agents used in ancient treatment systems may have therapeutic potential for many diseases. This potential is easily overlooked in an era of high technology medicine and heavy use of prescription medication.

This book has many unique facets. It traces the history of medical concepts from the ancient to the modern, but casts light on the repeated reinvention of the medical wheel. Few things are new in medicine. With major breakthroughs, what often occurs is a serendipitous discovery of mechanisms of action for beneficial medical interventions.

The authors argue against the nihilism that characterizes the fight between the alternative and the conventional medical community. Like it or not, the age of "pluralistic medicine"—to quote Dr. Holt—has emerged. He rejects the dichotomy in medicine that beleaguers the alternative and conventional medical practitioner, teacher, or researcher.

The chapter on the home use of herbal remedies is packed with useful advice, and broad classes of useful herbs are enumerated. In order to illustrate the promise of herbal therapies, Dr. Holt and Ms. Comac have used the example of the herb *Andrographis paniculata*. The use of this herb has often been reported in folklore, and it has a long history in Ayurvedic and traditional Chinese medicine. To take a single herb as an example and illustrate the steps in its pathway of research and development is very illuminating. Of great significance is the authors' discussion of the use of modern biotechnology research, such as signal transduction technology, in defining a scientific basis for the use of herbal extracts such as andrographis.

The book is written in a manner that will appeal to both the health care professional and the lay reader. It is a must for all health care givers who wish to satisfy their patients' ever-increasing desire to discuss natural medicines, herbal remedies, and botanical therapies. The knowledge it contains is highly relevant and timely in modern health care.

Thomas V. Taylor, M.D., FRCS
Professor and Chief of General Surgery
V.A. Hospital, Baylor College of Medicine
Houston, Texas

Preface

The Western medical establishment today is mired in controversy. Contemporary problems include skyrocketing costs, the effects of managed care (beneficial and adverse), inequities in the delivery of health care, ethical dilemmas — the list goes on and on! As the list grows, more and more people — health care practitioners and the public in general — argue the merits of alternative or holistic medicine as compared to "traditional" or allopathic medicine.

Everyone is tired of being told that medicine is "at the crossroads." Unfortunately, this crossroad has no traffic lights and there are good and bad drivers coming from both directions. Standard medical teaching has concentrated on the high technology approach with a quest for "wonder drugs." This approach has been at the expense of considering general public health measures and more natural options to prevent or treat disease.

The allopathic way is to reject a medical intervention if its action is not explicable in terms of current scientific knowledge, but this rejection does not take into account the inadequacies of that knowledge. The alternative health care giver, however, does not live in a perfect world. For every stubborn allopathic physician, there may well be a "wacko" alternative practitioner.

This problem in the direction of health care has been precipitated by patients' disenchantment with many conventional medical interventions. The modern patient has greater knowledge and new self-reliance. Many individuals want to engage in their own health care decisions, and consumers of health care have exhibited a much greater tendency to self-diagnose, self-medicate, and question their physicians. We are not judgemental; it is just that many conventional medical practitioners show an unwillingness to address their patients' newfound needs and demands. A solution may be at hand.

ix

This solution may rest in a meeting of minds in which health care givers can be more tolerant of each other's opinions. Joint preoccupation should rest in an obsession with what works rather than what is more palatable to the prevailing body of opinion. In a quest for conciliation, some have introduced terms like *integrated medicine* or *complementary medicine*. These labels do not help, because they foster the notion of a dichotomy of medical thought and opinion. In the next millennium, "good" health care will be pluralistic in its approach. The term *pluralistic* encompasses the idea that only what works and what is most sensible may be applied. Pluralistic medicine implies that a health care giver will take the trouble to become enlightened in modern medicine and more traditional or ancient medical systems. These earlier systems, which often use natural options such as botanicals, may have a lot to offer.

This book is about the use of herbs in health care. Mankind is not a stranger to herbs, but modern medicine has only just begun to reexamine their health-giving potential. The reasons for this delay in exploring the miracle of herbs are many. Such reasons are mostly rooted in the economic interests that so often drive political and social direction.

The political lobby rests with large corporations that must engage in self-interest. Multinational pharmaceutical industries support the lion's share of research in most medical institutions. Millions of dollars are spent on a trial to show that proprietary drug x is better than y. In this process the lateral thinker may be scorned, researchers often wind up in institutions that attract financial backing, and the researcher who puts his head above the pulpit risks being beaten over the head with the Bible! The authors of this book describe a revolution against this intellectual oppression. Hopefully, an increasing level of tolerance for research into natural remedies will develop. Herbs may have more to offer than the next poison pill for cancer chemotherapy.

On the one hand, proponents of alternatives such as herbal supplements extol their therapeutic value with the ardor of zealots. Opponents label those who defend such supplements as charlatans, quacks, and self-interested scoundrels. Resolving the controversy becomes increasingly difficult as misinformation, marketing propaganda, and stubbornness cloud the issue. Nevertheless, the "miracle herbs" are upon us.

Thanks to advances in molecular biology, biochemistry, and technology, the means to verify the therapeutic claims made for various herbs is at hand. Now cynics, skeptics, and believers alike will be able to avail themselves of the best nature has to offer.

We begin *Miracle Herbs* with a very brief look at the history of the healing arts — Western medicine, traditional Chinese medicine, and Ayurvedic medicine from India. You will learn that, all across the globe, herbs have played a major role in medicine since the beginning of time. You will also find out what happened in the West to change that.

In Chapter 2, you will discover how the healing arts once practiced by witch doctors developed into the medical sciences that include organ transplants, open heart surgery, and biotechnology.

In Chapter 3, you will see how — despite its glorious achievements — Western medicine has left many people dissatisfied. Many have turned away from the big business atmosphere that now surrounds the healing arts and have embraced a more holistic approach as well as alternative medications, such as herbs.

We will tell you how herbal medicine is tied to the fields of ethnobotany and chemical ecology. We will look at how and why herbs have come into prominence again. You will soon see that the renaissance in herbal medicine is just the tip of the leaf. A new era of medical miracles is being ushered in by the marriage of modern technology and ancient herbs.

In Chapter 4, you will learn all about the amazing new technique of "signal transduction" and the promise it holds for investigating novel drug therapies. You will also see how the technology can increase understanding about the biopharmaceutical effects of botanicals.

In Chapter 5, we will examine some of the reasons that scientists, physicians, and laymen believe that herbs can be used to treat disease. You will come to understand why herbs used by the Chinese, Native Americans, and South American Indians have long lured explorers, profiteers, and researchers into the forests and fields.

In Chapter 6, you will learn that some amazing discoveries are being made about botanicals that have been used in traditional medicine for centuries. You will find out how these herbs now promise to solve many of the medical problems that plague modern man. Herbs can, in fact, be used to treat everything from the common cold to diptheria.

Then, in chapters 7 through 9, you will discover exactly how signal transduction technology is being used to uncover amazing treatments for cancer, heart disease, and AIDS.

In Chapter 10, you will find a comprehensive listing of specific herbs and the ailments they can treat. The jargon used by people involved with herbals is also defined. In Chapter 11, you will get specific information on buying, preparing, and using therapeutic herbs. We give you hints on how to find the most reliable herbs and provide the names, addresses, and telephone numbers of various suppliers and information resources. Part of the chapter is devoted to the unique requirements of traditional Chinese medicine.

At the end of the book is a glossary defining all specific terms used. You will also find an annotated bibliography and a list of references. Appendix A includes technical data related to the scientific investigation of herbs, and Appendix B is a reprint of an article about the consequences of the 1994 Dietary Supplement Health and Education Act (DSHEA).

As we approach the twenty-first century, herbs may be the miracle that provides the answer to many of the dilemmas that assail twentieth-century medicine. Thanks to ancient herbs, the common cold, AIDS, cancer, heart disease, and other ailments may be vanquished.

Introduction

Modern science and technology are in the fast lane. Complex procedures such as organ transplants, in vitro fertilization, and cloning have moved into the field of medicine like a speeding train. Medicine is no longer an art practiced by physicians whose sense of touch, smell, and even taste must tell all. Today, the understanding of diseases has moved from the external signs to the most internal, right down to the molecular level.

The influence of high technology on medicine is not all good. Over the past fifty years, it has been responsible for a change in the practice of medicine: Talking to patients has become passé; the history and physical examination have been replaced by a blood test, an X ray, or a nuclear medicine scan.

To our benefit, however, modern science now affords us a way of testing folkloric tales that involve traditional remedies of natural origin. As the century closes, medical science is poised to explain the secrets of nature, revealing the secrets of health and disease. Mother Nature gave us remedies for most ills, and many have been discovered by serendipity or empiricism. Many are ancient and overlooked, and many are botanical in origin.

Modern pharmacotherapy has achieved a great deal in disease treatment, but it has also contributed to ill health. Synthetic drugs are overused, inappropriately used and, on occasion, held to false expectations. Never in the history of mankind has iatrogenic disease (health care–giver induced) been so ubiquitous. Inappropriate use of over-the-counter drugs for common ailments has become a public health concern of a magnitude equal to illegal drug use.

For example, the use of aspirin and nonsteroidal anti-inflammatory drugs are the most common cause of adverse effects reported to the Food and Drug Administration or other regulatory agencies in Western societies. Many people admitted to hospitals with life-threatening gastrointestinal bleeding are there because of the use of various ibuprofen and aspirin products. These drugs are often used to treat arthritis, but they only produce temporary relief and do not cure the underlying disorder. It is therefore no surprise that individuals may seek gentler, safer options for arthritis. This circumstance is reinforced by the success of the book *The Arthritis Cure* by Jason Theodasakis. This book discusses natural options for bone and joint health, but the data are not novel.

Those who suffer from chronic degenerative diseases desperately seek solutions, and natural herbal options do exist. Many of these have been used in medical systems for thousands of years. While millions of dollars go to develop the next patented, synthetic drug, the secrets of the ancient herbalists remain unlocked.

Nevertheless, interest in the medicinal use of herbs has increased. In fact, interest in ancient and natural or "alternative" remedies has burgeoned in recent years. You can't open a magazine or turn on the TV without finding mention of at least one natural remedy. Millions of unit doses of melatonin, shark cartilage, ginkgo biloba, and garlic have been consumed as dietary supplements with consistent, but not universal, reports of success without side effects. The market for herbs and dietary supplements has literally exploded.

Interviewed by *Newsweek* in 1995, William Watts, president of the health store chain General Nutrition Center (GNC), said, "I've never seen the momentum for the industry as strong as it is right now." Throughout the dietary supplement industry, sales of herbal remedies now exceed $1.5 billion each year, and GNC opened a new store almost every day for three years.

The use of dietary supplements is reaching epidemic proportions in the United States. The industry is now regulated to some degree by the Dietary Supplement Health Education Act of 1994. Despite the impending promise of regulation, many dietary supplement manufacturers are purveying products with health claims that cannot be substantiated. Unfortunately, the dietary supplement industry has not shown a willingness to police itself. Such practices broaden the gap between alternative and allopathic health care.

You may be surprised to know that sales of dietary supplements (or natural remedies) have been increasing in Southeast Asia even more rapidly than in the United States. For example, the Korean market for dietary supplements is estimated at $1.4 billion — and Korea has approximately one-seventh the population of the United States.

According to New York City's commissioner of consumer affairs, growth in the American dietary supplement market "far exceeds growth in the traditional drug market." It seems that Americans' veneration of scientific, conventional, or allopathic medicine is slipping.

As early as 1983, the *London Times* reported that the failings of modern medicine were fueling the alternative medicine movement. By 1992, research conducted by Harvard Medical School indicated that two-thirds of Americans used some form of alternative health care. Another survey indicated that 34 percent of patients — or 61 million Americans — had used at least one unconventional therapy.

What has fueled the movement? Skyrocketing medical costs and health insurance woes have certainly played a role. In an environment where medicine is a business and the general practitioner is a fading memory, consumers of health care services are seeking more control over their health and bodies. Recent research has repeatedly indicated that some of the most feared diseases — cancer, heart disease, and stroke — are brought on by our adverse lifestyles. Diet, environment, exercise, and freedom from stress are increasingly seen as crucial factors in health, factors for which the individual is solely responsible. People now believe it is in their power to improve their health and increase their longevity, so self-help books and books on alternative health care abound.

In addition, the American public has become increasingly concerned with ecology and more interested in using environmentally friendly products. Disillusionment with conventional medicine's inability to control cancer, AIDS, or heart disease — despite the billions spent on research — has perhaps played a larger role. Killer diseases in Western society remain unchecked: The AIDS epidemic has grown; the numbers of women dying of heart attacks has increased; the American Cancer Society continues to predict that by the year 2000 one of every two Americans will develop cancer.

Treatments for AIDS have been introduced but are prohibitively expensive. "Cocktails" of antiviral drugs for AIDS therapy have been touted with early reports of great benefit. Unfortunately, the AIDS virus has now revealed its recalcitrance and versatility, demonstrating that the cocktails are not as effective as had been supposed. The HIV virus can "hide" in memory cells in the immune system of its host. Intervention limitations and victims of HIV disease are growing as is criticism of the drug-approval process. Regulatory agencies are being blamed for slow approval of new therapies or for suppression of promising alternative botanical therapies.

Conventional therapy has not had a satisfactory impact on heart disease — the number one killer. Angioplasty had been touted as a revolution in the treatment of heart conditions, but its failure rate soon became well known. The limitations of angioplasty provide an example of the continuing disenchantment with conventional medicine.

Cancer treatments — surgery, chemotherapy, and radiation — continue to be applied in circumstances where they have little effect. On occasion, these interventions can maim and sicken patients. No wonder Americans are seeking a better way.

In seeking new solutions, Americans began to look at age-old treatments. Consequently, Ayurvedic medicine, the ancient healing system from India; traditional Chinese medicine; and rain forest botanicals are being investigated. Herbs, poultices, and tonics have been used around the world for centuries to cure ailments, boost immunity, and increase vigor. A question that repeatedly arises is: "Would these remedies have endured if they had no effectiveness?"

Interest in alternative medicines has escalated and is fed by fires fanned by the media. The public is deluged with reports about the powers of vitamins A and C, folic acid, melatonin, and garlic. Many claims of efficacy may have transcended scientific proof, but news reports generated increased demand for natural products. Thus, it was "only natural" that manufacturers, entrepreneurs, and promoters would see the profit to be garnered from alternative medicine. More and more products and services have become available and are advertised more heavily, as consumers have become increasingly interested.

Inevitably, the establishment realized alternative medicine would not go away if it were simply ignored. In 1992, Congress funded the Office of Alternative Medicine "to evaluate alternative or unconventional medical treatments." Some health maintenance organizations (HMOs) integrated alternative medical strategies with allopathic medical practices and found a concomitant lowering of the overall cost of health care. In many cases, there was also an increase in patient satisfaction.

Striking events have occurred even in countries with socialized medicine. In the United Kingdom, the demand for alternative treatment and homeopathic resources in the National Health Service has swamped the few clinics that had been set up to provide such services.

The option of natural medicinals is not, however, without problems. Varro Taylor, Ph.D., a retired Purdue University pharmacognosist (an expert in the medicinal uses of herbs), feels that consumers are being deluged with misinformation. In his opinion, some products may be worthless, and others can be downright dangerous. The purveyance of herbs and dietary supplements is not "actively" regulated by any government agency. There is often a passive "approval" process with occasional attacks on both unscrupulous and well-intentioned practitioners or suppliers of complementary medical treatments. Thus, the consumer has no assurance that a product is potent, pure, or even safe.

The danger of herbs has been emphasized by the recent deaths of several young people who were getting high on pills containing ephedrine or ephedra, derived from the *ma huang* plant. The tragedies led to attempts at consumer protection through legislation. The state of New York took the lead, but others have been slow to follow.

Is it possible to find out which natural medicinals are, indeed, effective? How can we find out whether an herb is safe? Can we learn which herbs are the most useful and the safest? In an effort to answer these questions, care givers, scientists, and representatives from the dietary supplement industry met in Washington, D.C., in the fall of 1996. They began to plan a "national formulary" to ensure authoritative standards and information sources for natural remedies.

It is surprising that the United States, with its prowess in modern medicine, has been so slow to develop standards for herbal or botanical remedies. One might speculate that the "consumerization" of Western society has stood in the way of progress, since the economic balance has rested with multinational pharmaceutical companies and the purveyance of synthetic, branded, or proprietary medicines.

Several European countries have taken a lead in the standardization and quality control of medicinal herbs. Germany and the United Kingdom have taken the initiative to develop herbal pharmacopoeias in recognition of the increasing public demand for herbal remedies. Recently, the British herbal pharmacopoeia has expanded to contain monographs on 169 medicinal herbs, and in 1996, eighty-five monographs were added. Some consideration should be given to the content of monographs on herbal medicine.

In herbal pharmacopoeias, herbs are identified by their pharmaceutical names and binomial Latin names. It is important to describe the characteristics of herbal medicines so that some standardization and consistency can be maintained among herbal products available to the general public. Quantitative methods of chemical analysis are also important in assuring consistency and, in turn, a reasonably predictable and reproducible biological effect. Unfortunately, there are still no clear guidelines for the quantitative assessment of active ingredients, and this uncertainty will have to be overcome to some degree by clinical trials that can measure dose response relationships, clinical efficacy, and tolerability.

An important new bridge in the gap of standardization of herbal or botanical remedies is the application of in vitro laboratory studies. These use the techniques of molecular biology and other biotechnologies to assist in identifying putative treatment agents and predicting their in vivo effects. For instance, it is possible to test herbal remedies' effects on various signals within cells. This field of study, known as signal transduction, looks at the way information moves from the nucleus of a cell to its surface. The information being passed plays a role in the development of inflammation and disease.

Herbal remedies are, therefore, being investigated with the aid of signal transduction assay systems. These enable researchers to test whether substances like herbs interfere with signals within cells. (Signal transduction technology is discussed in detail in later chapters of this book.)

Until now, we have had to rely on anecdotal evidence. Today's herbal books and alternative "how to's" describe what various people have done and experienced, but this kind of evidence has often been rejected by the medical establishment and by government agencies. Anyone who wants to have a drug approved by the Food and Drug Administration (FDA) has to go through a protracted process of animal testing before trying the drug on people. Each potential product has to be tested for toxicity, effectiveness, and optimum dosing before it can receive approval. Because this procedure is expensive, manufacturers only want to produce synthetic drugs for which they can hold a patent. Furthermore, manufacturers are frustrated by the problems of standardizing natural drugs; biologicals vary from batch to batch just as apples, bananas, and oranges do.

An apple is an apple and not an orange; however, an apple from Canada may resemble one from the United States, but the apples may have different tastes or nutrient qualities. The assumption that categories of dietary supplements are homogeneous or equally beneficial in their biological effects is grossly overlooked by consumers, health care givers and regulatory agencies. The dietary supplement industry is guilty of taking collateral information obtained from one specific type of dietary supplement and using it to generically support the sale of a product of the same category, even though it may not be identical in its efficacy or safety.

Examples of this type of misbranding are numerous and are not taken into account by the organizations that have evolved from the 1994 Dietary Supplement and Health Education Act in the United States. (Appendix B provides a lay account of the act, which is a complex piece of legislation with far-reaching consequences for the producers, consumers, and regulators of dietary supplements.) For example, an herbal therapy such as echinacea is used by thousands of consumers with the assumption that "echinacea" is effective in the treatment of colds and flu. Few consumers ever consider the type of echinacea they are taking, but the root of this herb has more active components than the stem or leaf, and there are probably major differences in biological effects. Also, the species of *Echinacea — angostafolia* or *purpurea —* differ in composition.

Research may be used to support echinacea's promotion of a certain biological function, but the research was done with a specific extract presented in a specific formulation in a discrete dose given at specific intervals. The idea that all echinacea is health-giving is naive, and the use of data derived from one type of echinacea to promote another is misleading. If done knowingly, such promotion could be construed as consumer fraud. Individuals who are interested in using botanical supplements (or herbal medicines) should therefore examine the scientific platform upon which a product is promoted.

An unscrupulous dietary supplement manufacturer may use inferior ingredients in a brand of a popular dietary supplement. In fact, this practice may be quite common. Manufacturers have sometimes falsely claimed that their manufacturing process enhances a category of natural remedy. The alternative health care community has a core of "non-licensed" health practitioners who may say anything to sell a dietary supplement product, and these individuals have no fear of reprisal from the authorities that control licensed practitioners of medicine, homeopathy, osteopathic medicine, or naturopathic medicine.

In the 1960s and 1970s, farsighted individuals in Europe recognized that monographs on plant drugs were frequently removed from official European pharmacopoeias. In recent times, this trend has reversed, due largely to the efforts of a few individuals and organizations that have had to work on a voluntary basis or, at best, with meager government support. It is interesting to speculate why systematic deletion of plant drugs and herbals has occurred. The process seemed to coincide with the emerging domination of multinational pharmaceutical companies.

After major drug discoveries were made in the 1940s and 1950s, drug companies furthered their own interests by using economic and political power to shape medicine. If a pharmaceutical company had a synthetic drug to sell, its interests were not served by a readily available natural remedy. Even though a natural remedy or herbal medicine may have been effective or cheaper than a synthetic, in the drug company's perception the natural remedy was merely "competitive."

The modern physician has been accused of having a well-lubricated prescription pen, and the quick stroke of this pen may have become too frequent. Many common ailments may be readily amenable to a natural option. Numerous times, the overprescription of synthetic drugs or the inappropriate use of over-the-counter synthetic medications has untoward or adverse effects.

A striking example of overuse of prescription medications in the face of effective natural interventions is the treatment of high blood cholesterol. A worldwide preoccupation with high cholesterol has created a multibillion dollar market for synthetic lipid-lowering drugs that may have questionable safety profiles. Some physicians have been willing to prescribe drugs to lower even modest increases in blood cholesterol, although the benefit of therapy is questionable and the risk-to-benefit ratio is not easy to assess.

Furthermore, these drug-prescribing practices have sometimes occurred in the absence of even nominal advice on lifestyle changes that can effectively reduce modest increases in cholesterol. Pharmaceutical companies have argued that clinical research demonstrates benefit, including a reduction in the risk of heart attack and death from coronary artery disease. These optimistic conclusions are hotly debated.

While this controversy occupies contemporary medical thinking, physicians have failed to acknowledge some botanical agents that have been shown to be safe, effective, and inexpensive in the treatment of high blood cholesterol. For example, soy protein in an appropriate formulation and quantity has been reported to lower blood cholesterol with the therapeutic equivalence of many synthetic cholesterol-lowering drugs.

The evidence of soy's benefit in this instance is overwhelming. In fact, in 1995 the *New England Journal of Medicine* published a statistical study of four decades of research on soy's cholesterol-lowering effects. Despite the prominence of this report by Dr. James Anderson and his colleagues from the University of Kentucky, the conventional medical profession has not even paid lip service to the news. Physicians continue to prescribe lipid-lowering drugs that are extraordinarily expensive and associated with onerous side effects, such as muscle damage and liver problems.

Meanwhile, practitioners of nutritional or natural medicine have been effectively using a dietary supplement called Genista — soy protein containing isoflavones. The cost-effective supplement has successfully lowered blood cholesterol without a single recorded side effect. In traditional Chinese medicine, soy has been used for centuries as an herbal remedy and food staple. This "secret" of the Chinese herbalist has now been revealed, but therapeutic use of soy seems inhibited by unclear influences.

Although accusations of paranoia within the complementary medicine community abound, a pernicious and powerful conspiracy appears to exist. These forces prevent remedies of natural origin from being applied as effective, first-line, cost-effective medical interventions.

Medicine in the Modern Age

About the time of World War II, the synthetic drugs penicillin and chloroquine (used to treat malaria) took the medical world by storm. The pharmaceutical industry began to grow and prosper. Prescription drugs and synthetic medicines became increasingly popular, and the use of medicinal herbs diminished so much that we often forget that herbs (plants used medicinally or as spices) gave rise to many modern pharmaceuticals. Drugs as common as aspirin (methyl salicylate), digitalis, and pseudoephedrine were all derived from botanicals. In fact, 25 percent of the pharmaceuticals sold between 1962 and 1973 contained at least one ingredient that was derived from plant sources. Today, the pattern has changed to the almost exclusive use of synthetic medicines.

The use of synthetic drugs is but one of many changes in the practice of medicine. Up until the end of the twelfth century, medicine was more art than science. It was not based on very exact knowledge: Traditional physicians often acted on instinct; the only means they had for checking their conclusions were the writings of the ancients. According to medical historian Benjamin Lee Gordon, M.D., F.I.C.S., author of *Medicine Throughout Antiquity* and *Medieval and Renaissance Medicine,* early physicians practiced medicine by "collating ancient opinion." They saw no need for devising any other tools or techniques. They proceeded without any clinical devices: no lab tests, no blood pressure gauges, not even a thermometer. Their only tools were their five senses.

Gradually, the practice of medicine began to acquire a more scientific basis. People began to reject astrology and superstition. They stopped turning to their gardens for medicines and headed, instead, to the apothecary shops. By the middle of the nineteenth century, pharmacology, the study of the changes produced in people and animals through the use of chemical substances, had entered the world of medicine.

Eventually, the pharmaceutical industry was joined by the biotechnology industry, which has enjoyed tremendous growth in recent years as a result of James Watson and Francis Crick's 1953 description of the structure and operation of the DNA molecule. With this discovery, our understanding of life mushroomed, leading ultimately to the development of genetic engineering. In this procedure, scientists can alter a living organism's genetic material to produce an organism with different characteristics than its parents.

Watson and Crick's discovery probably had as much of an impact on academia as it did on science, medicine, and industry. As the century progressed, scientists in academic institutions played a major role in emerging biotechnology companies: Genentech, Biogen, BioTime, Paracelsian, and Shaman Pharmaceuticals were formed by university professors and entrepreneurs who saw their commercial potential. In fact, in 1984, almost four hundred academic scientists were involved in 20 percent of the publicly held biotechnology companies. Billions of dollars are being poured into these companies, and many lay men and women are reaping large profits from trading in biotechnology stocks. Biotechnology companies have created an impressive collection of products, including a growth hormone; recombinant Factor VIII, a vitally important blood clotting agent; and bacteria that can produce human insulin.

The world of biotechnology, however, involves more than the manipulation of genes. Anytime microorganisms or biological substances are used for industrial or manufacturing processes, biotechnology is at work. This includes the use of yeasts in baking and wine making, and the bioconversion of organic wastes. Now a new field of biotechnology promises to revolutionize medicine.

Signal Transduction Technology

The life of every organism depends on a virtual cascade of biochemical processes, which occur within cells in response to a vast array of stimuli — internal or external. Various messages are delivered to the cells in a process referred to as signal transduction, the study of which is opening new vistas in biological and medical research.

Researchers have made great progress in identifying the molecules that control the cell cycle, which culminates in cell division. They also know that when the signals controlling the process are interfered with, a number of apparently unrelated diseases can develop. With signal transduction technology, these researchers can detect molecular changes associated with disease even before overt manifestations or symptoms appear. This technology has created a whole new era of investigation in pharmaceutical development.

At research laboratories in Cold Spring Harbor, for instance, scientists are studying two classes of enzymes, one that turns on and one that turns off a process critical to regulating cell growth, in order to better understand the role these enzymes play in disease. With this knowledge, they hope to ultimately develop drugs that will be effective in treating cancer, leukemia, diabetes, and perhaps some neurological disorders.

Meanwhile, at Tularik, a biotechnology company in San Francisco, scientists are already attempting to create signal-transduction-based pills. Much of the company's work is based on the identification of a molecule that signals more than one hundred different genes to inaugurate processes related to immunity and inflammation.

Scientists at a dozen U.S. companies are now using signal transduction technology to identify and measure the precise effects of synthetic and natural chemicals on cell division. The technology may soon play a key role in the development of dietary supplements. The leaders in this field are Paracelsian Inc., BioTherapies Inc., and Shaman Pharmaceuticals. For the first time, research in basic science will be used to test the efficacy of traditional and botanical medicines in vitro — in artificial environments outside a living organism.

This may be the most significant advance in the formulation of dietary supplements since the inception of the industry two decades ago. The application of this technology to the study of dietary supplements' potential role will go a long way in rebutting the rejection of these agents by conventional medical opinion. If it is possible to validate a botanical's effect on molecular processes such as signal transduction in cells, then a scientific basis for the use of supplements can be proposed, and this will support the folkloric use of those products.

Currently, it takes up to twenty years and costs more than $230 million before a drug can be made available to the public. With signal transduction technology, the time and costs can be radically reduced. By looking at changes on a molecular level, signal transduction technology will assist in verifying the therapeutic and prophylactic effects of various substances, which will also help to eliminate years of animal testing.

Because the Dietary Supplement Health Education Act of 1994 permits herbal extracts to be marketed as dietary supplements without FDA approval, a product can be on the shelves within nine to twelve months of its discovery. Such speedy development assumes that results in signal transduction experiments are valid predictors of in vivo health benefits.

In an era in which Americans have been looking back to natural medicinals to solve their problems, signal transduction technology will help them move forward. Two proteins involved in separate cellular signal transduction pathways have already been formatted into products for the detection of cancer, the identification of cancer-causing chemicals, and the discovery of anti-cancer drugs. A storehouse of traditional herbs is currently being investigated by Paracelsian, Inc., through signal transduction technology. The study is revealing natural compounds with properties that suggest that they could be highly effective medicines.

Recent studies of botanicals that have been screened in signal transduction assays have suggested that several ancient herbs can be used effectively in the fight against heart disease, cancer, and — perhaps most dramatically — AIDS. Not only are these some of the most debilitating diseases known, they are also diseases for which current therapies are far from ideal.

Surgery, drugs, and radiation — convention treatments that maim and sicken patients — have led many to seek more natural alternatives, but their search has often been thwarted by government agencies and the medical establishment. Advocates of natural or alternative medicine often claim that these groups squelch natural alternatives in their pursuit of greater profit. On the other hand, the medical and scientific establishment claims that advocates of alternative medicine are, at best, inferior scientists whose claims are not substantiated or, at worst, quacks and charlatans.

Neither group appears particularly open-minded, and both are too easily incited to angry words and name-calling. So vehemently are opinions expressed that public confrontations, including pugilistic behavior, have been recorded among advocates of conventional and alternative strategies. The book *Dirty Medicine* has drawn attention to these unfortunate confrontations among health care givers with polar viewpoints. As usual, the truth can probably be found somewhere in the middle.

Signal transduction technology should give both camps unequivocal answers. By providing scientific evidence to substantiate claims made for natural medicinals, signal transduction technology may satisfy proponents of both alternative and conventional medicine. The technology will also enable manufacturers to standardize herbals. In the process of standardization, it is necessary to identify the active component of the plant extract, and signal transduction experiments permit measurement of dose response data on molecular changes in cells. Different formulations or concentrations of plant extracts can therefore be studied. Paracelsian, Inc., has performed such work on extracts of traditional Chinese herbal medicines derived from their proprietary reference library of herbal extracts. Unfortunately, signal transduction technology may not be useful in ascertaining safety, which is best measured by human toxicological observations.

Thanks to signal transduction technology, the practice of modern medicine will be enhanced by the best of ancient herbal remedies. In coming years, physicians may find themselves studying — in the words of Edgar Allen Poe — "many a quaint and curious volume of forgotten lore." As the twenty-first century unfolds, biotechnology will form a bridge between the world of pure science and the purely natural world.

A Note to the Reader

The authors of this book are not attempting to provide advice on the treatment or prevention of disease. Dietary supplements are not to be used to diagnose, prevent, or treat any disease. This book was not written to endorse the use of any products — natural or synthetic — for any treatment purpose or health benefit. The conclusions represent the authors' opinions of medical, scientific, folkloric, and lay writings on the various health care topics discussed.

The publishers and the authors accept no responsibility for the use of any agents mentioned in this book. Before an individual self-medicates, he or she is advised to seek the advice of a qualified health care professional.

1

A History of the Healing Arts

From shaman to radiologist, the story of medical history is almost as long as civilization itself. This story can best be told as a saga of discovery, with mankind learning ever more about anatomy, drugs, hygiene, and microorganisms.

The story of the healing arts probably begins with plant medicines. Around the time of the cave dwellers, healers began to find therapeutic herbs through their "dowsing" instinct. In so doing, they were following the lead of animals who instinctively know which plants provide nutrition and which are poisonous. Consider that Indian wild boars and Mexican pigs ardently devour certain local plants that are known to be anthelminthic, or worm-fighting, and that there are many reports of chimpanzees and baboons eating leaves with known medicinal properties despite the unpleasant taste of the leaves.

In addition to instinct, traditional healers relied on their powers of observation, coupled with trial and error. They would use a botanical in different situations and watch for results. Careful note would be made of the plants that could induce bowel eliminations or urine flow, or of those with tranquilizing effects. The healers' ability to provide the appropriate botanical assured them a special place in society, and among healers, the shaman was paramount.

The word *shaman* derives from Tungus, a Siberian language, and indicates a man who understands the mysteries of life and death. It is believed that alone among priests, magicians, and witch doctors, the shaman can ascend to heaven or descend to the underworld.

The reign of the shaman, however, was relatively short-lived. Time passed. Religious convictions changed. The Church rose to power. All that remained of the lore of the shaman were his plant medicines. Yet herbs were not the only therapy used by primitive healers. The earliest medical procedure was probably cranial trepanning, in which primitive men would

1

open the skull roof to drive out the spirits that were causing disease. Evidence of the procedure survives in human skulls that show bone scars around the edges of the hole. Many patients survived this crude surgical intervention. Indeed, the scars attest to the patient's survival long after the operation.

Trepanned skulls found in ancient Inca settlements are taken as evidence of early neurosurgery for head injuries and intracranial bleeding caused in battle. Archaeological evidence also reveals that the early Egyptians were accomplished surgeons, but surgery in ancient Egypt may actually have begun as a death technique learned from the practice of embalming. Believing that the dead person's spirit would die if the body rotted, the Egyptians sought means to preserve the flesh. The complicated ritual of cleansing, stuffing, and wrapping involved in embalming began with the removal of internal organs, which were preserved and stored in jars. The embalming and preservation of mummies was made possible by the early Egyptians' skilled use of herbs and spices.

The Egyptians, however, were not the only ancients who knew about surgery. In India around 700 B.C., the Ayurveda, a comprehensive medical text, described a variety of surgical instruments that complemented the herbal formulary. Indian physicians apparently performed many operations on the stomach and bladder, and could even remove cataracts. Their skills as plastic surgeons were notable, as they frequently rebuilt wounded parts of the body, using hair to stitch up torn skin. The Chinese were the first to use anesthesia in the form of acupuncture to relieve the pain of surgery. We are not, however, certain who performed the surgery.

In ancient times, witch doctors, priests, and physicians competed with one another, each attempting to provide a rather one-sided interpretation of the mysteries of the human body. Priest-doctors in Eastern Europe then began to conduct medical experiments, records of which eventually reached Greece, where the first known medical school was established on the island of Cos in about 600 B.C. Hippocrates, known as the Father of Medicine, was born here in approximately 460 B.C.

The works of Hippocrates suppose that living bodies are composed of four humors: blood, yellow bile, black bile, and phlegm. Health was the result of the proper mix of these humors, and diseases were categorized according to the humor in excess. Perhaps more importantly, Hippocrates described a method of diagnosis based on observation and reasoning.

Among his most famous precepts are, "First, do no harm...Desperate diseases need desperate remedies," and "One man's meat is another man's poison." Ideas such as these spawned what is known as Hippocratic medicine, today's conventional or allopathic Western medicine.

About 500 B.C., Alcmaeon, a Greek living in southern Italy, began to dissect animals and compiled an anatomy book. In the second century A.D., Galen, a native of Asia Minor who became the physician to the Roman emperor, also performed dissections on animals, particularly the Barbary ape. As a result, Galen described the structure of animals and studied the function of their organs. His work was so respected that for ages, no alterations or corrections to his writings were permitted; his word was law in European medical thinking for 1,500 years. The esteem in which Galen was held may be due in part to his religious convictions. Though he did not convert to Christianity, he did believe in one God, and as the power of the Church grew during the Middle Ages, Galen's work gained preeminence.

Galen's work included descriptions of plants presented in an orderly scheme. His scheme established a division between the professional physician and the traditional healer, since the latter's frame of reference was based solely on a plant's observed action. Through their observations, traditional healers had come to expect that herbs would not work quickly; they were well aware that nature could not be hurried.

Because they had reference to Galen, however, professional "doctors" believed they had superior knowledge and could speed the healing process. The healing arts soon turned to active intervention in bodily processes. Bloodletting and purging to rid the body of excess humours became the order of the day. At the same time, the ancient scientific pursuits that Rome had prized were disappearing, as Rome's energies were directed to governing the empire. Scientific experimentation languished and was replaced by the preparation of manuscript herbals.

In the seventh century, the Arabs took over North Africa and became supreme in the Mediterranean world. Greek and Roman texts were translated and provided a basis for the flourishing of Arabic medicine. The Arabs established teaching hospitals, emphasized environmental factors in sickness, investigated disease at the clinical level, and studied preventive medicine and public health. One of the most eminent Arab physicians was Ar-Razi (865–925). Known as Rhazes in the West, he emphasized diet and hygiene in place of drugs: "Avoid complex remedies where simple ones will suffice," he wrote.

In the following century, Ibn Butlan claimed that clean air, moderate diet, rest, exercise, and a balanced emotional state were essential to health. It was perhaps Ibn Said, known as Avicenna (980–1037), however, who had the most profound influence on Western medicine.

A physician in Baghdad by the time he was seventeen, Avicenna had a passion for order and tended to be inflexible. A devout Muslim, he believed that God had provided medicine for all men's ills and actively investigated numerous botanicals. Thanks to his work, hundreds of herbs from places as far off as Persia, India, and the Far East were added to the *materia medica*. The plethora of herbs helped to make pharmacies a viable business, and in the ninth century the first stores opened in Baghdad. By the tenth century, Arab ideas were passing into Europe through Salerno, Italy.

The compounding of medicines, an extremely lucrative Arab business, was a major contribution of the time. Among the exotic newcomers were many cathartics and laxatives, which were essential to the practice of ridding the body of excess humours. The most important among these were senna (*Cassia acutifolia*) and rhubarb (*Rheum palmatum*). Imported from Turkey, this herb was found to be very effective against infectious diarrhea.

An eastern Mediterranean plant called scammony (*Convolvulus scammonia*) was often used as a purge or cathartic. Many considered the herb too irritating to use safely. The Arabs made it more reliable by boiling it in a quince, throwing away the scammony, and mixing the quince pulp with the seeds of psyllium (*Plantago psyllium*). The most common ingredient in bulk-producing laxatives today, psyllium is an annual Eurasian plant whose seeds provide soluble fiber. Although regarded as a modern medicine, it is merely a reinvention of the wheel.

Preparations such as these helped the apothecary trade grow, since apothecaries could not have made a living simply by selling what anyone could grow in his garden. The new compounds also helped physicians prosper. Doctors could now convince people that only they were sufficiently trained to deal with the complexities and perils of herbal medicines. A medical catastrophe of unbelievable proportions was required to initiate the next chapter in the Western world's practice of medicine.

The Growth of Medical Science

The bubonic plague swept over Europe in the mid-1300s, killing one quarter of the population. When the epidemic had passed, new hygienic and sanitary measures were established. Leper houses and general hospitals were built, but many did not seek out the new facilities. They believed that the plague had been caused by the unusual conjunction of Saturn, Jupiter, and Mars, which occurred on March 20, 1345. Furthermore, the seeming failure of the physicians to aid the dying led many people to believe they might as well do it themselves. The use of homegrown herbs abounded, and ignorance ruled.

Little was known about anatomy or the mechanisms of disease because research on corpses was prohibited at this time. It took almost two hundred years, until the height of the Renaissance, before the science of anatomy would flourish. The fledgling science owed much to Leonardo Da Vinci. Using scientific methodology, Da Vinci investigated the body and shared his knowledge through finely executed and detailed drawings. Sharing of information increased dramatically when Latin became an international language and the printing press was invented — and there was much to share, including one surgeon's technique for stopping bleeding by tying off blood vessels.

As the power of the Church diminished, experimentation and dissection increased, and so the seventeenth century became the age of physiology. Thanks to the work of Michele Servetus in Spain, Andrea Cesalpino in Italy, and William Harvey in England, the circulation of blood in the body was finally understood. An invention that is credited to both Zacharias Janssen and Galileo Galilei made its first appearance around the turn of the seventeenth century; it was called a microscope. Using this instrument, Marcello Malpighi soon observed that organisms were made of tissues and each tissue was made of "saccules," or cells. Cell biology would henceforth play a leading role in science. Subsequently, the Dutch scientist Van Leeuwenhoek discovered microscopic life forms, opening the door to the science of microbiology.

At the beginning of the eighteenth century, Giovanni Battista Morgagni conducted extensive studies of anatomy and repeatedly compared clinical symptoms with the organic changes he found in cadavers. He described the differences between healthy and diseased organs, thus spawning the science of pathology. The combination of these developments fostered medicine as well as science and helped encourage the creation of schools of medicine. In the United States, medical schools opened at the College of Philadelphia in 1765 and at Harvard University in 1782. These schools were offshoots of European medicine, with special influence from British medicine that emanated from the University of Edinburgh in Scotland and several medical schools in London.

American medical students were soon to have a drug of incalcuable benefit in their arsenal. An English physician, Sir William Jenner, discovered that small doses of cowpox injected in a human could provide immunity against smallpox. He first used the vaccine on an eight-year-old English boy in 1796, and it was introduced to America in 1800 when Benjamin Waterhouse vaccinated his son and six other members of his household. Two years later, President Thomas Jefferson vaccinated more than seventy members of his household, and use of the vaccination spread throughout the United States. Acceptance of the vaccine paved the way for the science of immunology. Eventually people would be immunized against a number of diseases when they were injected with specially treated germs or the serum fraction of blood from animals that had immunity.

In the nineteenth century, a Frenchman named Marie Francois Xavier Bichat advanced the science of histology, the study of normal and diseased cells. His work helped to confirm the theory that living organisms passed disease from one person to another. Thus the priest-doctor's role in medicine had come to an end. Shamans and witch doctors were considered powerless against diseases: No evil eye nor demon spirit need be cast out. The effort to control the spread of microorganisms would now become central to the field of medicine.

Microbiology Revolutionizes Medicine

By the middle of the nineteenth century, the Italian anatomist Filippo Pacini had described the first microorganism specifically associated with a disease — *Vibrio comma,* the microbe that caused cholera. Progress in microbiology, spearheaded by Louis Pasteur, would soon revolutionize the world of medicine.

A chemist who studied fermentation, Pasteur attributed this process to the presence of microorganisms and confirmed his theory through rigorous experimentation. He also produced incontestable evidence that microbes do not arise spontaneously from decaying material but breed from microorganisms that had been present in the material all along. He is probably best known for perfecting a process that kills bacteria responsible for tuberculosis and typhoid, and delays spoilage by killing other bacteria. This process is, of course, pasteurization.

Pasteur is considered a major player in the development of the germ theory of disease. According to this theory, diseases are caused by infectious microorganisms. With Pasteur's identification of several disease-causing agents, mankind began to conceive the possibility that disease was caused by a concrete if invisible enemy that could be fought.

The germ theory of disease led people to realize that sanitation and hygiene were necessary to managing the spread of disease. By the nineteenth century, public health was becoming a field of medicine in the United States. John H. Griscom studied tenement conditions in New York City in 1845, and Lemuel Shattuck conducted similar studies in Massachusetts in 1850. In 1866, Stephen Smith authored the New York Metropolitan Health Law. In 1869, Massachusetts became the first state to have a permanent board of health.

Shortly after this, Abraham Jacobi, M.D., of New York, regarded as the founder of American pediatrics, said, "Questions of public hygiene and medicine are both professional and social. Thus every physician is by destiny a political being...a citizen of the commonwealth with many rights and great responsibilities."

Meanwhile, a French scientist named Claude Bernard was espousing another point of view. Known as the Father of Experimental Medicine, Bernard believed that a person's internal environment was more important in determining disease than was the germ itself. He believed that the best way to deal with infectious diseases was to strengthen the body's own defenses. His theories were supported by a Russian scientist named Elie Metchnikoff, who had been deputy director of the Pasteur Institute in 1904. Metchnikoff introduced the theory of phagocytosis, the belief that some white blood cells can destroy harmful invaders. He also developed the theory that certain bacteria in the human digestive tract could prolong life by preventing putrefaction. Though largely debunked, this theory has reemerged in recent years with the increasing use of probiotics (friendly bacteria) that are available as dietary supplements.

Modern medicine has, for the most part, emphasized the role of germs and the synthetic battle against them to the exclusion of nature's defenses, which begin within the body. This emphasis took firm hold with the work of German bacteriologist Robert Koch.

Koch was able to isolate microbes and keep them alive in artificial media. By inoculating animals with those isolated organisms, he proved beyond a doubt that diseases are transmitted from one animal or person to another by a specific organism we now call a pathogen. In 1876, he discovered the microorganism that causes anthrax and subsequently uncovered the germs responsible for wound infections, conjunctivitis, and Asiatic cholera, among others. Having isolated the cause of tuberculosis, Koch attempted to discover a treatment. He developed a remedy based on a substance called tuberculin; this sterile liquid contains proteins removed from culture of the bacteria responsible for the disease.

Reviewing milestones in the history of medicine helps us recognize that advances in the treatment of disease — even if short-term — lead to radical changes in the body of medical opinion. While these advances have brought progress, radical changes in medical opinion have repeatedly resulted in the rejection of useful interventions from earlier medical systems. Medical opinion often falls into this trap when a single significant failure of a medical system results in rejection of the entire treatment system. Its useful components must then be rediscovered. The more one delves into the history of medicine, the more one realizes that physicians are constantly engaged in the reinvention of forgotten but sometimes highly effective remedies. This is the story of herbal medicine as we turn the clock of the new millennium.

The Growth of Chemotherapy

As scientists found out more and more about microorganisms and disease, they became convinced that effective weapons against specific organisms could be formulated. Sometimes immunization was an option, sometimes it wasn't. The "sickening" effects of some attempts at immunization led to the use of the term *inoculation*. The disguise was meant to convince people that the act of inoculation was innocuous — but this wasn't always true.

In any event, people continued to get sick, and there were no more incantations to bring them relief. So the science of chemotherapy was born. With chemotherapy, diseases are treated with drugs based on chemicals that have accurately defined structures.

In 1883, the German chemist Ludwig Knorr developed antipyrine, a synthetic compound that reduced fevers and deadened pain. A huge money-maker as well as the first completely man-made drug, antipyrine was one of the main agents that launched the synthetic drug business.

Industrial chemists in Germany feverishly sought to duplicate, or at least imitate, the product. Eighteen centuries after Dioscorides had recommended a decoction of white willow bark for gout, scientists discovered that the salicin in the bark gave it pain-killing properties. The synthetic form — salicylic acid — could not be used internally. Felix Hoffman of the Friedrich Bayer company began to test compounds of the acid for pain-killing and fever-reducing properties and discovered the astonishing effectiveness of acetylsalicylic acid — aspirin. A century later, aspirin is probably the most widely used drug in the world. It is estimated that more than one hundred million pounds are consumed each year to kill pain, treat rheumatoid arthritis, and prevent blood clots. Despite this phenomenon, it is Paul Ehrlich who is often credited as the father of chemotherapy.

It was Ehrlich who first sought a "magic bullet" — a substance that could modify diseased tissue without affecting healthy tissue. His research revolved around the use of arsenic to treat syphilis. In 1910, Ehrlich's 606th arsenic compound proved to have low toxicity and high specificity against *Spirocheta pallida* (*Treponema pallidum*), the agent that causes syphilis. In the early 1930s, sulfa drugs were developed, and chemotherapy entered its golden age. Sulfanilamides were used to fight such pathogens as streptococci and staphylococci. The first sulfanilamide was Prontosil, which was derived by Gerhard Domagk, a German researcher, from a quick-acting red dye for wools; the dye was originally synthesized by Paul Gelmo, an Austrian industrial chemist. Domagk subsequently used

Prontosil on rats that had been injected with fatal doses of streptococci. The rats survived, and Prontosil was soon being used worldwide without regard for its adverse effects.

Even before that — in 1928 to be exact — Alexander Fleming had chanced upon a colony of mold that halted the growth of staphylococci in a petrie dish. The mold belonged to the species *Penicillium notatum*. At that time, interest in the substance was slight at best. During World War II the infection-related mortality rate was astronomical — even with the sulfa drugs — so research into penicillin began in earnest. During the first five months of commercial production in 1943, four hundred million units of penicillin came out of the factories. By the end of 1948, more than eight million *million* units were being produced — and so began modern man's dependence on synthetic drugs.

Pharmacy turned its back on the plant kingdom for several reasons. Many in the medical profession pointed out that plants had never provided an adequate remedy for syphilis, but synthetic drugs had. Furthermore, it was a synthetic — penicillin — that finally put a brake on infection. Then, too, plants were not likely to provide medicines that could be patented and marketed with a good profit margin. The growing pharmaceutical industry relied ever more heavily on synthetic drugs — sometimes foolishly so, as demonstrated by a study conducted at Metropolitan Hospital in New York City.

In 1918, 1,082 tuberculosis patients at the hospital were treated with every known therapy and with garlic. Dr. W. Minchin reported, "Garlic gave us our best results," but his work was ignored, and tuberculosis remained a killer disease. Then, in 1941, an article in *Science* pointed out, "researchers dealing with plant medicinals are relatively rare and are becoming more so... Present-day medical scientists only too frequently are apt to look askance at those who would investigate the therapeutic possibilities of the vegetable kingdom." Things have not changed since 1941, as evidenced by the frequent victimization of alternative medical practitioners by regulatory agencies and licensing authorities.

Using More Than the Five Senses

As the twentieth century unfolded, the death knell was sounded for herbal medicine. The skills of the herbalists and traditional healers — instinct, powers of observation, a special "healing touch" — were disappearing too. However, the isolation of the East, especially China, permitted the practice of traditional medical systems to flourish. In the West, by the beginning of the twentieth century a whole new chapter in medicine was being written.

The German physicist Wilhelm Roentgen discovered what he called X rays, which passed through the flesh of his hand but not the bones. The image of the skeletal hand could be captured on a photographic plate. Doctors the world over now had a way of actually seeing *inside* the human body. Thus, technology and medicine merged to present the world with the first miracle in diagnosis. Radiology soon played a role in treatment, too: Pierre and Marie Curie found that X rays and rays emitted by radium could be used to destroy tumor cells.

Now that the door to scientific medicine was wide open, men of genius were not content with examining the tiniest life forms or the internal workings of the body; even the workings of the mind had to be understood. Prior to World War I, the Austrian doctor Sigmund Freud delved into the hidden corners of the mind, and his ideas about the conscious and subconscious began to spread. Freud believed that neurotic symptoms and illnesses were caused by the need for suppressed emotions to find relief. Discussions between doctor and patient — known as psychoanalysis — could help the patient relieve the pent-up emotions in a healthy way.

Freud's belief that the mind and body are one, with mental factors influencing physical ones, opened a new vista in the treatment of mental illness, and the medical field of psychiatry was born. Despite Freud's preoccupation with mental dynamics, he had a keen interest in herbal medicine, including, but not limited to, his own addiction to cocaine.

Today, psychoanalysis, behavior modification, and drugs work together to cure the ills of the mind. Although drug use is relatively new to the field of psychiatry, pills and potions pervade Western medicine. Still, drugs are not the only tool used by today's health care practitioners. A veritable treasure chest of medical instruments and procedures is available.

Technology and Medicine Join Forces

We've obviously come a long way since shamans drilled holes in people's skulls to let out evil spirits. Today, chemicals, radiation, and surgery combat microorganisms, system malfunctions, and even molecular abnormalities. Modern medicine benefits from a plethora of sophisticated techniques and high-tech equipment. Many of the medical sciences spawned before the twentieth century bore fruit in this century because of burgeoning technology.

One of the earliest technological advances was the electron microscope, which brought scientists into contact with the smallest units of which life is composed. The study of biochemistry now investigates the basic processes of life, molecule by molecule. New chapters in medicine will tell the story of chemical phenomena that take place deep within us and are at the root of disease. These chapters will continue to rely heavily on technology.

Biotechnology in Historical Perspective

Biotechnology is not new. When the first hunters and gatherers began to plant crops and domesticate animals, they were using biological organisms to fulfill their needs. Crop rotation, selective breeding, and the creation of hybrid plants are probably the best known uses of biotechnology. The technological innovations of the twentieth century, however, moved us far beyond Gregor Mendel's laws of inheritance. Today, biotechnology permits us to alter the very stuff of life to fulfil our needs and desires. We can actually harness life processes and put them to work in commerce and industry.

The era of biotechnology probably started in 1953 with James Watson and Francis Crick's description of the structure and operation of the DNA (deoxyribonucleic acid) molecule. Their discovery moved biotechnology away from farmers and into America's research laboratories and universities. Because of the discovery, our understanding of life mushroomed, leading ultimately to the development of genetic engineering. This technology permits researchers to develop organisms or cells whose offspring have genetic combinations that were not present in the parents. Ideally, genetic engineering can be used to eliminate genetically transmitted diseases such as Huntington's chorea and Down's syndrome. Till that day dawns, bioengineering is making other medical advances.

Before genetic engineering, therapeutic or prophylactic substances that exist in the human body were available only on a limited basis. Companies had to extract the substance — a hormone — from a bodily fluid or from ground organ or gland tissues. Obviously, obtaining sufficient material was an expensive and arduous task for both purveyor and producer.

Take the example of Premarin. A hormone replacement therapy used in mature menopausal females, Premarin is derived from the urine of pregnant horses. In addition to being repugnant to many women, the therapy involves the harassment of pregnant horses. Use of the drug continues, even though modern research demonstrates that plant compounds can effectively reduce menopausal symptoms. Phytochemicals such as phytoestrogen from soy (PhytoEst) have been shown to alleviate hot flashes and assist in promoting cardiovascular health and bone structure, important issues in the menopausal female.

To provide two year's worth of the naturally occurring growth hormone absent in dwarfs requires fifty to one hundred pituitary glands, which are taken from autopsied cadavers, whose numbers have become increasingly scarce. The hormone, therefore, had to be rationed until synthetic alternatives became available. In addition, extracts from the pig pancreas have traditionally supplied the insulin used to treat diabetics. Recombinant DNA technology led to the development of a bioengineered growth hormone and bacteria genetically engineered to produce human insulin.

Recombinant Factor VIII is a vitally important blood clotting agent. Because hemophiliacs lack this agent, a simple cut can cause them to bleed to death. There is also a genetically engineered vaccine for hepatitis-B. Interferon, an antiviral used to battle cancer, is another result of biotechnology, as are microbes that can pump oil from wells and transform industrial pollutants into energy sources. According to science writers Sharon and Kathleen McAuliffe, "Genetic engineering holds such power that it is often called biological alchemy — a way of turning DNA into gold."

DNA, the chemical that carries genetic information, can now be removed from one organism, attached to the DNA of another, and made to work within the second organism. DNA contains regulatory information that controls when a gene is turned on or off and when a protein will be synthesized.Each gene on the DNA chain is unique for a single protein. Each protein is a chain of molecules that has a characteristic size and shape and carries out one function. Hormones are proteins. Enzymes, the catalysts that slow down or speed up chemical reactions in our body, are proteins. Hemoglobin is also a protein, as is collagen, the main constituent of skin. Antibodies are proteins, too.

In 1971, Paul Berg of Stanford University was the first to construct a recombinant molecule, for which he earned a Nobel Prize in 1980. In 1973, Stanley Cohen of Stanford and Herbert Boyer at the University of San Francisco first transferred a recombinant molecule into a living organism.

In June 1980, a Supreme Court decision allowed researchers to patent genetically engineered life forms. Genetic engineering has received extensive media coverage, but other techniques are also being used. Cell fusion mixes the contents of cells that are unmateable, creating hybrid offspring. One of the techniques associated with this technology allows scientists to create monoclonal antibodies, specific antibodies that the body can use as weapons against foreign invaders and cancerous growths.

Another type of genetic engineering involves the transfer of foreign DNA into a cell via a virus. In this process, called transduction, target cells are removed, infected with a retroviral vector carrying a normal gene, and then returned to the patient. The vector virus is capable of only one infection because it does not have the information needed to make viral proteins.

One of the newest fields is signal transduction technology. In this field, investigators can "read" and intercept the biochemical messages related to control of the cell cycle. This technology will ultimately prove that many materials, including botanical agents, have molecular effects. Application of this technology will bring herbal medicines to a new era of respectability as their role in disease prevention and treatment becomes increasingly defined. Signal transduction technology will enable researchers to identify herbs that can halt molecular changes that cause illness. The anecdotal evidence so long scoffed at by scientists will no longer be the sole documentation for efficacy. Medicine now stands at the crossroads, as science shows no favor to traditional or alternative medicine.

Engineering Technology in Medicine

Although genetic engineering is a branch of biotechnology, both are radically different from biomedical engineering. In fact, college students who are interested in genetic engineering take biology and chemistry courses in a school of arts and sciences. College students who study bioengineering are enrolled in a school of engineering. Although they study biology and chemistry, they study engineering principles with an eye to the design of instrumentation and prostheses.

Diagnostic techniques have gained a great deal from advances in engineering technology. Following the invention of the X-ray machine in 1895, specific radio-opaque materials were developed that could outline organs of interest. Contrast media enables physicians to see blood flow patterns, permitting diagnosis of arterial blockages, pulmonary embolisms, and aneurysms.

Late in the 1950s, image intensifiers made it possible for cardiologists to see holes in heart walls, leaking valves, and the structure of the entire coronary artery system. Then the invention of the cyclotron allowed for the development of radioisotopes. These radioactive pharmaceuticals are used with gamma-ray detectors to trace radioactive emission from various tissues. The isotopes are used to check the functioning of the thyroid and liver, and to determine blood volume.

At the end of the 1970s, the computed tomography scanner — CT scanner for short — was perfected. During a CT scan, electronic signals from a revolving X-ray source reveal successive pictures of various body structures. The pictures today are so good that even an inexperienced eye can pick out various internal organs. Subsequent technological developments such as sonograms and laser dopplers have contributed to the revolution in diagnosis. Treatments involving heart-lung machines, organ transplants, and artificial body parts further demonstrate the extent to which technology has revolutionized medicine.

Modern Western medicine certainly seems more science and technology than art. In other parts of the world there are healing practices that have retained a sense of art and humanity in the skill of their practitioners. Many are attracted to these systems because, as author Christopher Hobbs puts it, "we want to connect the 'mind' of scientific understanding with the 'soul' of traditional medicine."

Traditional Chinese Medicine

In a world beset by stress and the health problems it engenders, traditional Chinese medicine — often referred to as TCM — can seem like an oasis. In

TCM, health depends upon a person's internal harmony and vitality. Traditionally, the people of China have embraced the spiritual world in lieu of the material. In the absence of the material, humankind turns to the spiritual and recognizes the satisfaction that can be derived from the environment. Chinese civilization is founded on Taoist tradition, and Chinese medicine is based on the same concepts of balance and harmony evident in Chinese arts and sciences. Of course, medical treatment is part of traditional Chinese medicine, but treatment is secondary to promoting health through lifestyle.

Ron Teeguarden, an author and former premed student who turned his attention to Eastern philosophy, writes of nine characteristics that are central to Tao philosophy and, therefore, to traditional Chinese medicine. The first is change, the recognition that there are no constants in life or in nature. Only Tao does not change. Because change is the one constant, flexibility is essential to the Way. Rigidity in nature leads to death. Therefore, another principle of life is adaptability.

We must be able to adjust to changes in the environment, just as a birch bends in the wind and does not break. After all, evolution is a process of adapting to a changing environment. If we are healthy, our bodies adapt to changes in temperature, light, and humidity. Goose pimples, dilating pupils, and perspiration are some of the ways the human body adapts to maintain homeostasis, or balance. A healthy person can adapt to and survive changes in external stimuli. If a person is unhealthy, he is less able to adapt and more likely to perish. In traditional Chinese medicine, tonic herbs enhance adaptability so that we can expand the borders of our environment.

Congruent to change is cyclicity, the process that gives order to change. It is a fundamental principle of life that all processes in nature are cyclical. The *I Ching*, a Chinese classic also known as *The Book of Changes*, breaks a cycle of change into sixty-four primary divisions. Many scientists today concur that there is a biological or circadian rhythm to life. Recognition of the cycles permits us to anticipate changes of mood, vulnerability to stress and illness, and response to medical treatment. The most fundamental rhythm of life may be the cell cycle, which can be assessed by signal transduction technology.

Just as the Bible says, "To every thing there is a season, and a time to every purpose under the heaven," the *Tao Te Ching* says:

> For all creatures there is a time of advancing,
> A time for withdrawal
> A time for inhaling, a time for exhaling,
> A time for growing strong, a time for decay.

In a world that is constantly swinging between extremes, balance is thought to be the secret of health and happiness. Times when hard labor is required must be balanced with periods of deep rest and relaxation. When life is tranquil, we need the balance provided by recreation. Finding balance is often instinctive. Even animals seek shade and cool liquids when it is hot. When it is cold, they seek a warm lair and hot drinks. A fundamental component of traditional Chinese medicine is herbal therapy, the application of which must fit the underlying philosophy of the way Chinese practice medicine. Some concepts are worthy of further review for the reader.

The philosophy of the Way, or Tao, obviously draws inspiration from the patterns of nature. The predominant pattern — the first law of the universe as we know it — is the principle of yin and yang. These represent the complementary poles in the universe; they are the two parts of any whole — e.g., top and bottom, front and back — which must be in balance.

When we conceive of a rhythmic shifting from one pole to its opposite, we are able to understand the concept of yin and yang, the fundamental pattern of all processes. Each process has a time at which energy must be accumulated and processed so it is usable; this phase is yin. Yin conserves. Each process has a phase in which the energy is expended; this expansive or active stage is yang. Yang radiates. Once the energy is expended, the entity or phenomena seeks new sources of energy, and so the cycle of yin and yang continues.

In medicine, one of the most graphic examples of this phenomenon occurs in the heart, where electrical energy flows through the nervous system into the A-V, or auriculo-ventricular node, which helps regulate the heart rate. This energy builds until the node is saturated. The accumulated energy is then discharged throughout the muscle, causing a strong contraction that forces blood out of the heart through the body. This yang phase is then followed by the yin stage of energy accumulation.

Yin and yang are often characterized by the Eight Entities, four pairs of characteristics, as seen in the following:

Yin	Yang
Cold	Hot
Deficiency	Excess
Internal	External

These entities are guides to physical conditions. A person with a hot condition experiences physiologic and metabolic hyperfunction. He or she will be nervous and overactive, easily agitated. When there is a condition of deficiency, vital energy is drained; one experiences exhaustion and hypofunctioning organs. The internal entity refers to the viscera.

The yang entity refers to the overall condition of the remaining yang energies. People with a cold condition have lessened physiological and metabolic functioning. They experience fatigue and sluggishness. When there is excess energy, the normal flow of energy is being blocked. People with this entity will appear strong and willful, have a strong and quick pulse and possibly an excessive libido. The external entity refers to the body's surface or skin.

The organs of the body also exist as complementary couples: the yin heart and the yang small intestine; the yin liver and the yang gallbladder. Each pair of coupled organs is governed by one of the Five Elemental Energies. The kidneys and bladder are, naturally, ruled by water energy, the heart by fire energy. When there is imbalance between the two poles, physical disorder results. If the fire energy of the heart is excessive, high blood pressure, heart palpitations, and a rapid pulse will probably result. Western medicine treats the heart to eliminate these symptoms.

In traditional Chinese medicine, the root cause is seen as a deficiency in kidney energy that created an imbalance. The kidneys are treated to increase water energy, which regains control over the heart's fire energy, and abnormal heart symptoms disappear. Some of these concepts are difficult to understand and represent a totally different pattern of thought than in conventional Western medicine. However, they form the basis of our understanding of herbal therapy in traditional Chinese medicine.

Herbs are also yin and yang. Yang herbs heat the system, stimulate organs, and accelerate metabolism. Yin herbs cool the system, calm vital organs, and slow internal energies. Diseases are treated with the appropriate herbs: Acute constipation is seen as a yang condition — hot — and is treated with yin — cooling herbs — such as rhubarb and aloe.

Practitioners of traditional Chinese medicine know which herbs have a natural affinity for which organs and energies. More than two thousand items are listed in the pharmacopoeias of China, but in practice only about three hundred are commonly used, and only one hundred of these are considered vital to formulating common prescriptions.

The modern physician in Western society and allopathic interests in Eastern medical culture do not concern themselves with yin and yang, but are preoccupied with the basis of the pharmacology herbals used in traditional Chinese medicine. Although they recognize the effectiveness of the herbs, they cannot understand the philosophy underlying their discovery and use.

Over several millennia of experience and observation, practitioners of traditional Chinese medicine have found herbs that can strengthen the body, increase fertility, and even prolong life. In the Orient there are many tales of Taoists who lived to extreme old age. One man, Li Ch'ing Yuen, is believed — even by modern scholars — to have attained the age of 252. Born in 1678, he set out from home at the age of eleven with three herb traders. The group traveled throughout China, Tibet, and Southeast Asia studying herbs and herbal traditions. It is said that Li consumed little meat, few root vegetables, and limited grains. He ate little more than herbs such as *Lycium chinensis*, *Panax Ginseng* combined with *Radix Polygonum multiflorum* and above-ground vegetables that were steamed. It is not a coincidence that many modern day antiaging remedies are rooted in traditional Chinese medicine.

The Chinese medical system also revolves around the concept of energy flow, or Qi. Pronounced "chee," and sometimes spelled chi or ch'i, the word means "life energy." Because Qi creates life, its management results in health and longevity. Disease occurs when Qi is blocked or flowing to excess; then there is a state of imbalance. Oriental scholars have long studied the means by which life energy can be managed. Various healing arts, such as yoga, resulted. Yoga practitioners discovered that energy runs through the body in a circuit known as the organ-meridian system. There is a set of points at which these energy circuits can be influenced by pressing, rubbing, and tapping. The arts of acupressure and acupuncture were developed.

It has been confirmed time and time again that there are points on the body, which when stimulated appropriately, provide anesthesia and/or analgesia — pain-relief without loss of consciousness. Western researchers now believe that endorphins — hormones with opiate characteristics found mainly in the brain — may come into play during acupuncture and acupressure. Further confirmation has come from studies involving Kirlian photography, which demonstrates that living substances radiate bioelectricity. In fact, it has been shown that people who have the proverbial "green thumb" radiate an energy that is beneficial to a plant's bio-field.

Qi meridians occur in yin and yang pairs, of which there are five: wood, fire, metal, water, and earth. Water is a state of extreme yin, a period of rest and quietude. Winter is of the water element because nature is indrawn. Water concentrates at the body's core, regulating the mineral balances, strengthening the bones, and nourishing the marrow.

Wood is the next phase. Concentrated energy explodes outward, initiating a period of activity. Spring is the corresponding energy. In the body, this energy is responsible for the drive to procreate. If sublimated, this energy can turn to frustration and anger. When this energy is depleted, lethargy and depression remain. Only when expressed and satisfied in harmony with natural laws is this form of energy properly nurtured.

Eventually the explosive power of wood levels out, and a sustainable high level of activity ensues. This is the fire stage. Energy is now expended freely. This phase corresponds to summer, when life flourishes. Fire is seen as the energy of growth, love, and compassion. It is the urge to care, give, and share. If this energy is blocked, tension, excitability, hysteria, insomnia, and nightmares result. If this energy is deficient, there is suspicion, paranoia, and memory loss. This is the phase of accumulation and storage.

When energy begins to be drawn inward, the metal stage occurs. Energy is less abundant than in the first stage and cannot be recklessly expended. The product is now being "harvested" and waste materials are being eliminated. If sufficient energy is stored, the process returns to the water stage. If insufficient energy is accumulated, the process runs out of energy and releases its stores back to nature. If we block the flow of this energy, grief and melancholy ensue. Breathing difficulties, impaired resistance, and dull skin can result.

Finally, there is an energy stage inherent in all the cycles: earth. This fifth energy represents the center and balance. In a human being, it is homeostasis, in which the earth element is always present and balance is preserved. Earth is the energy of memory and reflection. It nourishes and builds strength. When this energy is excessive, worry, obsession, hypochondria, and digestive, blood, and menstrual disorders occur. If it is deficient, the mind and body are heavy and sluggish.

Each of the five elements corresponds to a yin organ that is solid and a yang organ that is hollow, as seen in Table 1. If wood dries out when the sun is too hot, Qi is flowing from the wood to the fire. You can solve the problem by adding water to the wood. If someone's liver is overheated, a clinician can solve the problem by stimulating the kidneys; the liver is already too stimulated. A Western physician would say that by increasing the flow from the kidneys, toxins are eliminated.

TABLE 1
Elemental Associations of the Organs and Viscera

Energy	Element	Wood	Fire	Earth	Metal	Water
Yin	Organ	Liver	Heart	Spleen	Lungs	Kidneys
Yang	Hollow Viscera	Gallbladder	Small Intestine	Stomach	Large Intestine	Bladder

From the *Textbook of Advanced Herbology*, by Terry Willard, Ph.D., Calgary, Alberta, Canada: Wild Rose College of Natural Healing, 1992.

A Western practioner would also say that diseases are caused by microorganisms. A practitioner of traditional Chinese medicine says that a Qi pool has been created because the flow of Qi was blocked. This pool is a perfect habitat for microorganisms. In other words, the microorganism is not the cause of the disease but the result of the Qi pool. Restoring the proper flow of Qi will eliminate the microorganisms by eliminating their habitat; thus, the disease will be "cured."

Traditional Chinese medicine holds that the root cause of all disease is imbalance and deficiency in the internal energies that regulate the body. If imbalances are not corrected, serious malfunctions in biochemistry and internal organs occur. The malfunctions impede the immune system, permitting microorganisms to gain the upper hand. By the time symptoms have become apparent, the disease is very difficult to cure.

Practitioners of traditional Chinese medicine treat the patient, not the disease. These healers attempt to correct the imbalances through which disease entered. Because certain herbs have affinity for certain meridians, those herbs can be used to open the blockage along that meridian. The contemporary allopathic physician may balk at these concepts, which have been borne out by centuries of experience.

Traditional Chinese medicine reminds us that man is part of nature, dependant on the environment for support. Disease prevention and care are thus linked to nature. Man is subject to the laws of nature; violating them can cause illness. If man lives in harmony with the environment, life flourishes. More and more, modern Western society is discovering the truth of this principle. Our growing concern with ecology reflects our understanding that if we destroy the environment, we destroy ourselves. If water and air are polluted, we are poisoned. If the ozone layer is depleted, skin cancer rates increase.

The Chinese pursued the study of humankind's relationship with nature and have learned to use the resources of nature to develop "radiant health." Taoists especially employ tonic herbs and have developed their use to a sublime art. The masters, however, point out that it is Tao, through nature, that is the only healer.

Tao has two meanings: the absolute eternal nature of all being and non-being, and the Path or the Way. People follow the Path, or Tao, to eventually become one with the Great Tao, the Absolute-Eternal. Health-promotion arts such as yoga, meditation, Tai Ch'i Chuan, acupressure, and tonic herbalism are only temporary aids until one learns the truth about life and nature and is truly healed. Managed medical care could learn much from these ancient concepts.

Ayurvedic Medicine

The Indian subcontinent is the site of one of the oldest civilizations in the world. India had its beginnings around 2500 B.C. Since then, it has been overrun and controlled by various powers. Despite foreign influences, cultures unique to the Indian subcontinent continued to flourish, as did their multiple traditional medical systems. The British, who were in control from 1857 until 1947, learned much from East Indian folkloric medicine. In fact, traditional Indian medicine is widely practiced even today.

Ayurvedic medicine is one of the most famous Indian systems of medicine. The name Ayurvedic is derived from *Ayur* meaning "life" and *veda*, meaning "science." There are numerous similarities between Ayurvedic medicine and traditional Chinese medicine. It is of great significance that the two have many similarities but developed in isolation of each other.

In Ayurvedic medicine, as in traditional Chinese medicine, the basic energy of the universe has five components: ether (the space occupied by a cell), air, fire, water, and earth. These blend into three principles called *tridosha*. The underlying theory of *tridosha* is that health depends on maintaining a balance of the components. The *tridoshas* are individually known as *doshas*; these may be construed as mind-body types. The three *doshas* are *vata* — ether and air, *pitta* — fire and water, and *kapha* — water and earth.

Vata has the qualities of air, and therefore of movement. It governs such things as breathing, blinking, heartbeat, and contractions. It also governs catabolism, the internal process by which complex chemical compounds break down into simpler ones. During catabolism, energy is often released. The emotions that correspond to the *vata dosha* are nervousness, anxiety, and spasms. People with this *dosha* tend to be thin, distinctly tall or short, energetic, enthusiastic, and imaginative. *Vata* people crave sweets, sour and salty tastes, and hot drinks. This *dosha* is centered in the large intestine, pelvis, bones, skin, ears, and thighs.

Pitta has the energy of fire and heat. It governs metabolism, the sum of processes governing the breakdown and synthesis of nutrients to generate energy and maintain life. In addition, *pitta* governs temperature, intelligence, and understanding. The emotions associated with it are anger, hate, and jealousy.

Those with a *pitta dosha* are of medium height with a slender frame. They are well-spoken and intelligent, but tend to be irritable. They desire sweets, bitter and astringent tastes, and cold drinks. People with a *pitta dosha* avoid hard work, but like to possess and exhibit luxurious possessions. They would rather be leaders than followers.

Kapha draws from the water and earth; it is the cement of the body. People governed by *kapha* tend to be physically well developed. They have good stamina and physical endurance but are slow-paced and of a tranquil nature. They like pungent, bitter, and astringent foods. *Kapha* people tend to have great vitality. Their wit may be slow, but it is solid.

Kapha lubricates joints, provides skin moisture, and promotes wound healing. It governs strength, memory, and the energy of the heart and lungs. Greed and envy, forgiveness and love are the emotions associated with *kapha*. This *dosha* governs anabolism, which is the opposite of catabolism. During anabolism, nutritive matter is assimilated and converted into living substance.

As you can see, your *tridosha* governs your physiological and psychological functioning. Your *dosha* gives you specific emotional, physical, and mental tendencies. These ancient concepts are known to have a clear basis in scientific fact that has been discovered in the past fifty years of medical research.

Most people are not governed by a single *dosha*. A person can have one of seven constitutions with one or more of the *doshas* prominent:

1. *vata*
2. *pitta*
3. *kapha*
4. *vata-pitta*
5. *pitta-kapha*
6. *vata-kapha*
7. *vata-pitta-kapha*

The goal of Ayurvedic medicine is to balance the environment with personal constitution. The approach is holistic; mind and body are treated as a whole. When examining a patient, an Ayurvedic physician first establishes the patient's *dosha*, or mind-body type, through questioning and observation. Such things as pulse, eyes, tongue, nails, lips, sleep habits, and temperament will indicate the prevalent *dosha*.

For instance, a *vata* pulse is thready and feeble. A *pitta* pulse is moderate and jumpy, while a *kapha* pulse is broad and slow. Any imbalances are noted and then the physician attempts to restore balance. In Ayurvedic medicine, as in traditional Chinese medicine, the emphasis is on prevention. The goal is to check the signs regularly so that imbalances can be found early and easily corrected.

The *Charaka Samhita*, the "textbook of Ayurvedic medicine," discusses diet, exercise, enemas, and massage as therapies. Treatment programs usually begin with some program of detoxification. In addition, a great many herbal remedies are discussed. Ayurvedic herbs are categorized by taste (*rasa*), quality (*guna*), potency (*virya* or *veeya*), and the taste that arises after digestion (*vipaka*). *Rasa* can be sweet, sour, salty, pungent, bitter, or astringent. The qualities of herbs are arranged in ten pairs and include hot or cold, soft or hard, sharp or dull, heavy or light. Potency is categorized according to the particular *dosha* or *doshas* that an herb can pacify. In addition, potency refers to such actions as moistening, heating, purging, and increasing or decreasing specific secretions.

Today, Indian people visit a *vaidya*, one who can prescribe the herbs necessary to brew healing teas. *Kapha* tea is a stimulating tea that is traditionally taken when the weather is cold and wet. *Kapha* tea is considered beneficial for those who are overweight or lethargic. The cooling *pitta* tea is a hot-weather tea. It is recommended for those who are irritable or impatient and those with sensitive skin. The calming *vata* tea is taken when the weather is cold and wet. Those who are restless or stressed when traveling are said to benefit from this tea. It can also help those who have difficulty falling asleep or staying asleep throughout the night. (See Chapter 11 for sources of Ayurvedic teas or herbs.)

In these traditional medical systems, the botanical or herbal intervention alone may not achieve the desired health benefit without the holistic application of the medical system. Fortunately, modern medicine is approaching an understanding of holistic therapies, as evidenced by an increasing interest in lifestyle medicine, which is described in ancient medical systems. In medicine, nothing is "new."

Conclusion

As civilization progressed, people's belief in the influence of the stars and in evil spirits passed into obscurity. Scientific knowledge burgeoned. Technological advances seemed to make all things possible, and medicine became less art than science. It also seemed to become increasingly cold and impersonal. Gone was the relationship between patient, family, and practitioner. Gone, too, was the sense that there was healing power in a practitioner's special touch.

2

Conventional Medicine Today

Marcus Welby is no more. The drama of high-tech operations and frenzied emergency rooms on *E.R.* and *Chicago Hope* has replaced quiet pearls of wisdom. The image of the gray-haired family physician who arrived at your door, black bag in hand, has passed into folklore. Jack Kevorkian is here to represent our sense of desperation and social suicide. Strangely enough, Dr. Kevorkian is one of the few American physicians who still makes house calls.

Perhaps the old images have been driven off by the new concept of managed care with its cost-cutting mentality. Today, we're likely to believe that physicians are driven more by the profit motive than by a love of humanity. Bear in mind that there has been a systematic attempt to undermine the medical profession in many Western societies, and physicians have been their own worst enemies. However, while good physicians may be offering help and compassion to their patients, they are unforgiving and frequently vicious to each other. Perhaps their training and thoughts of perfection have molded this situation.

Health Care Becomes a Business

According to an article by Gary Stix in *Scientific American,* some people are experiencing "nostalgia for a more compassionate interaction between physician and patient, the antithesis of the managed care ethos. 'People get treated today as if they're a disease or an organ.'"

Herbert Benson, M.D., author of *The Relaxation Response* and a professor at Harvard Medical School, notes, "People are hungry for a better relationship with their doctor." Many believe that the doctor-patient relationship has been commandeered by managed care. The insurance companies and businessmen that run the HMOs do not offer compassion, hand-holding, or faith. Old-fashioned quality care has been replaced by the bottom line — how much does it cost?

According to the *Medical Herald*, managed care has significantly undermined the traditional doctor-patient relationship. The publication claims that the damage is so severe that many physicians are contemplating leaving the profession. One of the physicians quoted in the article is Richard Sanchez, M.D., chief executive officer of a physician practice management company called New York Doctors MSO. Dr. Sanchez says, "Physicians want change, especially primary care physicians, who are on the front lines of medicine and are feeling increasingly overburdened by paperwork, administration, and negotiating responsibilities under managed care." Practicing medicine in a managed care environment is not fun!

A survey of two hundred physicians in the New York area revealed that 45 percent believe managed care has had a negative impact on the quality of physician-patient relationships; 51 percent believe managed care has jeopardized their ability to exercise professional judgment; 47 percent believe the problem will get worse. Yet the practice of medicine today centers around managed care and its profit-driven businessmen. Approximately 57 percent of Americans now participate in a managed care health program; 17 percent have a "nonmanaged" health plan; the remainder are covered by a government plan like Medicare.

The number of caring doctors that are accused of overutilization, excessive billing, or unnecessary diagnostic testing is staggering. In community hospitals in managed care–intensive states, physician review organizations have left only a handful of physicians without a challenge to their recommendations for hospital admissions. Many of the doctor-watchers are clerical assistants, who are instructed to assess medical practice according to a recipe book. Their actions are driven by agencies that want to shift health care profit from care givers to corporate health care organizations. Profits in the not-for-profit hospital environment survive because of the strength of the hospital lobby. These are not cynical words. They are matters of fact.

HMOs are not the only problem in conventional medicine today. Many practitioners adhere to "scientific" medicine's emphasis on the human body as a machine like any other. So important is this doctrine that physicians were sometimes taught to treat a disease and not be swayed or distracted by their patients' feelings or opinions. In orthodox medicine, the physician's point of view is valued first and foremost, and the doctor is venerated as an expert.

The patient, on the other hand, appears not to be trusted. The patient is not always informed of all pertinent information, nor is he or she permitted to choose medicines or procedures. No wonder 70 percent of the three hundred physicians surveyed early in 1993 reported that trust between patient and physicians had declined during their careers.

The authors of this book are not members of the "doctor-bashing brigade." Quite to the contrary, we are ardent supporters of the majority of well-intentioned physicians who practice in a lousy medical environment that has been created by big business. Physicians are largely honest, ethical, hardworking individuals who are attempting to do their best. They are the product of their education, which espouses and defines unattainable standards.

Modern medical systems beckon profit but attempt to deny the providers of health care a decent living and a dignified environment. Lateral thinkers in medicine are often persecuted, even in our time of an individual's right of assertion. Some hospital administrators play a role in undermining the medical profession by engineering the program of managed care. Some salaries of hospital administrators in not-for-profit hospitals are obscene, and the profits being garnered by drug companies are no less astonishing.

Pharmaceuticals in the Twentieth Century

Modern American medicine may well be called the Age of the Pill. Since Paul Ehrlich began experimenting with chemical drugs in order to destroy the agents that caused diseases — in particular syphilis — chemotherapy has been a mainstay of medicine. In 1910, Ehrlich announced that his 606th arsenic compound was effective against syphilis, and people have been looking for a "magic bullet" ever since.

The dream of the elusive magic bullet was heightened in 1928 when British bacteriologist Sir Alexander Fleming discovered penicillin. Since then it's been, "Take a pill." Whether it's an antibiotic, aspirin, amphetamine, or tranquilizer, there's a pill for what ails you. There are literally thousands of drugs available to treat everything from a headache to obsessive-compulsive disorder to a heart attack. We keep believing that there will soon be a pill for the common cold, acne, the flu, and even cancer. Maybe this pill will be an herbal extract. The prevalence of drugs is not, of course, Fleming's fault; it is an example of the quantum leap prevalent in medical opinion.

Meanwhile, patients have developed a casual attitude about disease, believing that a pill can always cure their ills. As a result, they pay less attention to prevention. Yet prevention is often as simple as avoiding risks. Patient complacency has probably contributed to the development of drug-resistant strains of bacteria. Drug-resistance, one of the biggest problems in health care today, may be the result of excessive use of antibiotics. Patients continue to be all too eager to ask their physicians for them. Regardless of the nature of their condition — bacterial, viral, or psychosomatic — patients want to be cured the easy way. They want nothing more — or less — than a glass of water and an oblong or round tablet. Prozac has replaced the everyday pursuit of pleasure and is a crutch for happiness. The response from complementary medicine is to produce the natural product Nozac, which may not work!

Commonly seen in hospitals, antibiotic resistance is a dangerous problem that makes modern antibiotics useless. Consequently, infections such as tuberculosis are now much more difficult to treat, especially if they occur against the background of compromising forces such as stress or immune deficiency, as in AIDS. Today investigators are turning *away* from drugs in their attempt to defeat antibiotic resistance. At Yale University, for instance, researchers are trying to use enzymes found in bacteria to block the genes that provide drug resistance. This is a sign that cues from traditional medicine are at least fueling modern research protocols.

There is no doubt that synthetic pharmaceuticals save lives each minute of every day, but the chemical revolution has not been problem free. There are grave risks associated with incorrect dosing, medicating with too many drugs, drug allergies, and side effects. Consider that aspirin use by children can lead to Reye's syndrome, acetaminophen has been linked to liver and kidney damage, and ibuprofen can damage the liver and kidneys. Amoxicillin can cause nausea, vomiting, and diarrhea. The use of Minoxidil has been linked to headaches, dizziness, and urinary tract infections. Pick up any guide to pharmaceuticals and you will find a list of contraindications or side effects next to each and every item listed. Sometimes you will be horrified by the list of possible effects.

Statistics reveal that there are more than ten million adverse reactions to FDA-approved medications each year. Yet most people believe that if the FDA has approved a drug, it is safe. On the other hand, there is an unfortunate misconception concerning natural therapies. Some people erroneously presume that anything natural is safe. Consumers of herbal remedies must be aware that the most toxic compounds known to man are botanical in origin, and some commonly used herbs are highly toxic when misused. Just because something is natural, it is not necessarily safe.

The Role of the Food and Drug Administration

Established in 1931 as an arm of the Department of Agriculture, the Food and Drug Administration is an agency of the U.S. Department of Health, Education, and Welfare. It is charged with protecting the health of Americans. The FDA ensures that foods are pure and wholesome, safe to eat, and produced under sanitary conditions. Chemicals added to foods must be proven safe before they can be added. The FDA also sets limits on the amount of pesticide residues that can remain on crops. Labeling regulations for food, drugs, and dietary supplements attempt to guarantee honesty. A food is considered mislabeled if it is purported to fulfill a dietary need associated with a specific condition but the label does not support the claim. The label must include specific information about vitamin, mineral, and other dietary properties that the secretary of the FDA "determines and prescribes to be necessary in order to fully inform purchasers as to the food's value for such uses."

FDA regulations also address drugs. These are defined as articles that will be used in the treatment or prevention of disease in man or other animals, and "articles (other than food) intended to affect the structure of any function of the body of man or other animals." The agency makes sure that these drugs and therapeutic devices are safe and effective when used according to directions.

In addition, the FDA oversees cosmetics, making sure that they are harmless and made from appropriate ingredients. Coloring agents used in cosmetics, food, and drugs must be tested in FDA laboratories before they can be marketed. According to FDA regulations, drugs must be labeled and packaged honestly, and must include any warnings necessary for safe use. Representatives of the FDA inspect drug plants at least once every two years. If drugs are not deemed safe for self-treatment, they are restricted to sale by prescription.

Although Americans often speak of FDA bans or recalls, these are court actions that usually occur at the behest of the FDA, which then publicizes the recalls to make the public aware that a risk exists. The agency can also recommend that manufacturers or distributors withdraw a product.

In most circumstances, the FDA does a great job, but these are not small tasks. At times, the FDA is overwhelmed in its role of regulating and evaluating the safety of food and drugs.

In an attempt to minimize the dangers of drug use, the FDA has instituted a rigorous testing procedure. Drugs — articles designed for use in the diagnosis, cure, mitigation, treatment, or prevention of disease — require FDA approval prior to marketing. Filing for a new drug application requires at least two well-controlled clinical trials performed in multiple centers on several hundred patients.

An investigational new drug (IND) exemption, however, must be obtained from the FDA before human clinical trials can be conducted. The chemistry of the compound, as well as its strength, quality, and purity, must be investigated; it must be demonstrated that it is manufactured and controlled with "good manufacturing practices." The new drug approval process then involves evaluating safety (phase one) and efficacy (phase two) in humans.

People with chronic ailments and serious conditions, as well as lesser complaints such as headaches, allergies, and baldness, often volunteer to participate in clinical trials in order to gain access to therapies even before such help is available to the general public. Patients are referred by a doctor, must meet the medical criteria established in a specific protocol, and must be fully informed of any possible risk. In addition, participants receive care that is supervised by the government, is provided by extremely qualified practitioners, and is free of charge. Of course, it is possibile that a participant is not receiving the active drugs. Clinical trials usually involve control groups that receive placebos or standard drugs.

While clinical trials can lead to FDA approval for a drug, no such route exists for dietary supplements. The distinction between drugs and dietary supplements creates great problems. Sometimes a company marketing a dietary supplement attempts to conduct clinical trials to indicate a body structure function for which the supplement is sold. In this case, the FDA says, "You can't do that. If you do, you cannot maintain your status as a dietary supplement because you are a drug." At best, a dietary supplement can be labeled "misbranded" by the FDA. The system appears to present a catch-22 to manufacturers of dietary supplements.

On the one hand, manufacturers want to present the public with as much data as possible. The FDA may, however, view clinical trials of dietary supplements as investigations that require an investigational new drug exemption to continue. Once the company secures an IND, the compound is not considered a dietary supplement and must go the round of clinical trials to secure new drug approval. According to the FDA, a product that is publicly investigated or approved as a new drug before being marketed as a dietary supplement cannot subsequently be marketed as a supplement unless the FDA determines it is safe to do so.

It is not surprising that consumer groups, dietary supplement manufacturers, and innovative health care givers become upset or frightened by these restrictive regulations. Their concerns are compounded by a lack of clear guidelines. There are practically no precedents for the lawfulness of clinical trials of dietary supplements. Therefore, any trials are likely to be challenged if they serve as a basis for the promotion of the supplement, which then could be considered a misbranded drug. What a mess!

Herbal products today fall into the category of "dietary supplements." In the 1960s, as a result of the horrifying birth defects precipitated by the drug thalidomide, the FDA toughened its regulations regarding drug approval. At that time, certain widely used traditional medications were exempted from the testing requirements. Only a few of these were herbal medicines and included mint, which contains menthol, an approved treatment for respiratory congestion. Interestingly, mint is not very effective as a decongestant, but it is highly effective as a carminative or promoter of digestive relief. However, the FDA will not acknowledge the overwhelming evidence of peppermint as a safe and effective treatment for digestive problems such as bowel spasms or irritable bowel syndrome.

Dietary supplement manufacturers may not make any claims regarding herbs' therapeutic potential. If claims are made, the FDA fraud unit investigates and may have the product removed from the market. Retailers may also face the fraud unit if they display herbal products and literature lauding their medicinal value in close proximity to each other. A reprint of an article describing medical benefits constitutes a health claim if it is distributed with the product.

The Task Force on Dietary Supplements has recommended that herbs be regulated by the FDA as drugs. This would require that manufacturers subject the herbs to the same testing as any new pharmaceutical, a process that can take up to twenty years and cost over $200 million. Because herbs cannot be patented, no manufacturer would be willing to incur the expense, and herbs would disappear from the marketplace.

As interest in and investigation of alternative medicines has grown, it has become increasingly apparent that many nutriceuticals — naturally occurring agents that exert a positive influence in the human body — are valuable for maintaining health and resisting disease. Activists lobbied long and hard for a change, and in 1994 the Dietary Supplement Health and Education Act was passed as a result of pressure from many groups. This act recognizes that various minerals and botanicals can play a role in promoting health and in preventing diseases such as cancer, heart disease, and osteoporosis. Before the act was passed, various nutriceuticals — vitamins, minerals, fiber, garlic — were considered food or dietary supplements, not drugs. Because they were considered items to be added to particular foods or a person's diet, no medicinal claims could be made for them and they were controlled by the FDA's food regulations, not by regulations for drugs.

With enactment of the Dietary Supplement and Health Education Act, the labels on dietary supplements can now include statements regarding the substance's role in affecting body structure or function. The label can also characterize the documented mechanism by which an ingredient acts to maintain such structure or function. Labels can provide descriptions of general well-being resulting from consumption of the ingredient. The information must be substantiated and the labels must be truthful and not misleading. In addition, the FDA must be notified thirty days prior to the first appearance of the statement, and it must be accompanied — whether on the label or in ads — by the boldface message, "This statement has not been evaluated by the Food and Drug Administration. This product is not intended to diagnose, treat, cure, or prevent any disease."

The legislation exempts certain dietary ingredients on the market before October 15, 1994. If a dietary supplement contains an ingredient that was not on the market prior to that date, the FDA must receive evidence of a history of use or other evidence of safety at least seventy-five days before the product is to be marketed.

What's Wrong With the FDA

In the United States, the time and money required to secure FDA approval means that new drugs are slow to hit the market. Many believe that the FDA's approval process costs lives. The lay public, as well as physicians and scientists, have voiced strong criticisms. People who are ill want help as quickly as possible, and representatives of drug companies want to see a speedier review process in order to increase revenues.

One of the reasons for the high cost of drugs is that pharmaceutical companies incur great expense to get approval from the FDA. Obviously these companies have to recoup that expense if they are to stay in business. We all recognize the extremely high cost of brand name drugs, and many health care recipients have opted for the less expensive generic pharmaceuticals. Today, some insurance companies refuse to pay for brand name drugs if a generic equivalent is available, even if the generic drug may not be as good! Consumers have been duped by some generic pharmaceutical manufacturers who have been caught fudging data regarding their products' equivalence to brand name prescription drugs.

Although the FDA has streamlined its drug review times in recent years, the Pharmaceutical Research and Manufacturers of America (PhRMA) still feels that Americans must wait too long for new drugs to become available. PhRMA President Alan F. Homer actually claims that "the total time it takes to get the medicine from the lab into the pharmacy...is getting longer." His statement is based on studies indicating that the decrease in approval time has been canceled out by an increase in the time for clinical development. Between 1994 and 1995, the average time between the beginning of clinical trials and the completion of the application to market a drug was 7.2 years. Between 1990 and 1993, that time was 5.5 years.

Homer has also expressed concerns about a recent plan to improve the written labeling information on prescription medicines. Although he believes that written information is important to assure patients optimum benefit from their medications, he contends that the new system is too restrictive and emphasizes a drug's hazards rather than its benefits. In addition, the plan fails to recognize the role of the drug's providers and that of dispensing pharmacists.

Instead, it creates a new bureaucracy to administer the plan. The proposal requires pharmacies to supply necessary information. Pharmacists are thus forced to provide professional advisory service for which they are not reimbursed, imposing a financial burden without providing incentives to ensure compliance. This practice may have contributed to retail pharmacists' increasing interest in natural remedies such as dietary supplements, which have high profit margins and relativley low risk of liability. Pharmacists should be encouraged to take this pathway for the benefit of health care consumers.

Sometimes, it seems that the FDA is not doing as good a job as we might like. In 1973, for instance, Wyeth-Ayerst received approval to market the antiobesity drug fenfluramine. Sold under the brand name Pondimin, the drug was supposed to be used only by those who were significantly overweight — by 20 percent or more. In 1996, the FDA approved a new antiobesity drug, dexfenfluramine (sold as Redux). When fenfluramine is used along with phentermine, the combination is called Fen-Phen.

More than six million Americans have used Redux and Pondimin, but in July 1997, researchers at the Mayo Clinic reported thirty-three cases of heart valve defects in people taking these medications. In September of that year, the FDA analyzed the heart tests of 291 of the drugs' users and found that heart valves were damaged in almost one-third of them. In the general population, less than 1 percent have such damage. Subsequently, upon the recommendation of the FDA, Wyeth-Ayerst decided it would be "the most prudent course of action" to pull the drugs from the market.

It seems surprising that drugs with the side effects of Redux and Pondimin could have passed through the FDA approval process without their dangers being noted, yet at least one researcher had cautioned against approving the drugs. He said that if you give animals doses of the drugs sufficient to bring about weight loss, the animals suffer brain damage. One of the counterarguments was that the drugs had already been available in

Europe for a number of years without incident. We now know, however, that in Belgium there was some evidence of problems for years. No one had ever made the connection between the heart valve problems and the diet drug, or, if they had, their opinions were muffled.

Continuing questions about the FDA's ability to protect the public swirled around the diet drug issue even after the recall. Just days later, the FDA announced approval of yet another obesity drug — a combination of the previously approved phentermine and the antidepressant fluoxetine hydrochloride, or Prozac. Thomas Walden, Ph.D., an obesity expert, appeared on the television program *Good Morning America* and said it was "unconscionable" for the FDA to have approved the drug.

According to Dr. Walden, there had been little or no scientific testing of the new combination, and Prozac had never been approved for the treatment of obesity. Dr. Walden claimed that the manufacturer of Prozac had never sought approval because evidence of its role in obesity was "meager." In fact, in the *Nursing Drug Handbook*, anorexia, or loss of appetite, is not even listed as a possible side effect of Prozac, although that is a consideration with many drugs affecting the central nervous system. Although the FDA has approved a relatively untested synthetic, it has been unwilling to even consider granting approval to an herbal-based obesity drug. The herbal preparation is a combination of St. John's wort and *ma huang*, which contains ephedrine alkaloids. Some believe the reluctance stems from the deaths of college students who used ephedrine to get high and overdosed. However, ephedrine is a common ingredient in over-the-counter cold preparations and, in that form, has never been implicated in a fatality.

Prominent scientists and physicians have voiced skepticism about the FDA's efforts to help the public. According to Dr. Gerald Dermer, a staunch critic of current cancer research, the FDA approves poor or ineffective drugs — "virtually useless products" — because researchers are not presenting the agency with anything effective. Critics of the FDA also believe that the agency sometimes *hinders* the advancement of patient care. One such critic is Bert A. Loftman, M.D., who questions the role of the FDA in advancing an orthopedic technique called "spinal fusion."

Dr. Loftman has been questioning the FDA's relationship with the two major types of fusion instrumentation: pedicle screws and threaded cages. Some surgeons had been experimenting with the screws for years. Ten years ago, they applied to the FDA for approval. According to Dr. Loftman, "the FDA ignored them," but the surgeons continued to improve the device and the technique until its use became widespread. The FDA decided to consider the screws, halted educational courses that the researchers had been conducting, and initiated a study to see how well the screws worked. Physicians who had used the screws were then taken to court for having used a device that had not been approved by the FDA. Ultimately, the screws were found efficacious and were approved.

Has anyone paused to think about the losses and inconvenience of the physicians who were trying to do the best for their patients? These doctors faced sanctions and legal costs that might have ruined or seriously impeded their careers. Exoneration in these matters is not compensation.

In October 1997, after five years of evaluation, another device that aids the fusion of bones was approved by the FDA. According to FDA guidelines — known as the experimental protocol — neither the device (called a threaded cage) nor the technique for using it could be changed during the course of the evaluation. This appears foolish since it negates the possibility of improving the device as flaws become evident. Aren't clinical trials initiated to determine how a product functions in real settings?

Furthermore, the FDA will consider a study flawed and invalidate it if the mandated number of subjects is not reached or is exceeded, or if 85 percent of follow-up studies do not corroborate the results. As Dr. Loftman points out, "even if the cages were good, a flawed study would prevent their use. What of the patients that might have benefitted?"

Dr. Loftman believes that interference by the FDA is a violation of the Fourth and Tenth amendments in the Bill of Rights and claims that the agency delays and hinders the development of new treatments. He explains that an earlier method of using hooks to fuse the spine is inferior, yet is still approved by the FDA.

"The FDA is clearly counterproductive when it comes to efficacy," he writes in the February 1997 issue of the *Medical Herald*. "The older inferior methods drop by the wayside as the new methods advance. All of this can and should occur without government input...Setting the medical standards should be the province of patients and their doctors." This sounds appropriate, but the reality is that doctors are often no longer in control of their profession.

Some believe that the state of affairs at the FDA drives many Americans out of the country. They head to Western Europe in pursuit of drugs deemed "safe and efficacious" there but not in the United States. In Germany, for instance, health claims may be made for herbs so long as they have been proven to be safe and effective. Proving such efficacy in Germany is far less time-consuming and expensive than in the United States. Data can come from existing literature and anecdotal information from physicians. Clinical studies need not be extensive, and once an herb is approved, an insurance company will reimburse the cost if it is prescribed by a physician.

One editorial writer claims that the FDA is charged with keeping our medications safe, but is sometimes "guilty of excessive caution." Julian Whitaker, M.D., has a different slant on the issue. "Unfortunately, concern for public safety does not appear to be motivating the FDA's regulatory activism," writes Dr. Whitaker. "The FDA, in apparent collaboration with the drug companies, must find it profitable to keep us dependent upon manufactured, expensive drugs." The author of several popular books and founder of the Whitaker Wellness Institute, Inc., Dr. Whitaker had been trained as a surgeon, but soon turned his attention to preventive medicine and the use of natural remedies.

Pharmaceuticals Are Big Business

Governmental regulation is not the pharmaceutical industry's only problem. Public perceptions of the industry are not always favorable. Some people believe that pharmaceutical companies have switched many safe and efficacious prescription drugs to an over-the-counter status in response to people's desire for individual responsibility. Some view this switching of drugs as a political initiative to cut down on health-care costs. The switch will decrease patient visits to physicians for illnesses that are readily diagnosable and responsive to safe and effective remedies. Who lobbied for this political initiative? Perhaps the multinational pharmaceutical companies who stood to gain from enhanced brand-product life as patents expire on proprietary medicine.

The industry is often criticized for charging too much and for pressuring physicians into writing too many prescriptions. In a single year, drug companies expend approximately $600 million advertising prescription drugs. This money certainly seems to be spent in an effort to *create* demand for drugs, even if there is no obvious need.

The pharmaceutical industry is in the business of making money, and it does it well. In fact, it is the most profitable industry in the United States. Prices for prescription medication have been rising at four times the rate of inflation. Interestingly, the prices that seem to go up the most and the most frequently are for drugs used by baby boomers and the elderly, the largest consumers of drugs.

The costs of drugs for catastrophic illnesses are often astronomical. The average six-month supply of a cancer drug developed through biotechnology can cost more than $75,000, which may result in the loss of a life savings. Furthermore, the effect of this expensive therapy in most forms of "solid" cancer is of marginal benefit at best.

More than forty-five thousand sales representatives besiege American physicians in the attempt to convince them that their companies produce the best of all possible pills (vaccines are not considered lucrative). That works out to one sales rep for every twelve prescribing doctors. On the average, a physician will see two or three of these reps each week. Many doctors rely on these people as their primary and possibly only source of information about new drugs, but the sales reps and the literature disseminated by their companies are not confined to doctors' offices. Pharmacists, nurses, and hospital administrators are also deluged by information. It is not unusual to find sales reps hosting weekly luncheons at hospitals. In addition to lunch, the doctors and nurses receive pens, books, calendars, and other items imprinted with the company's logo and the names of various prescription drugs. It is estimated that the total cost of drug promotion exceeds $3 billion annually. The authors of this book have been grateful recipients of these minor inducements in their professional careers.

Physicians are busy with patients and a mountain of paperwork required by the government and insurance companies. Often they are hard-pressed to find time to keep up with the literature and the latest in scientific research. Consequently, they may find themselves writing prescriptions because a sales representative supplied them with information. Some prescriptions may be written because of a particularly memorable rep or a convincing sales pitch. Even the *Physicians' Desk Reference*, or *PDR*, the book physicians refer to most frequently, is not purely objective. Drug firms pay more than $12,000 a page to be listed in the book, which is mailed to doctors without charge. Few people, however, would blame a for-profit corporation for taking advantage of an opportunity to purvey its proprietary product.

The drug companies' influence seemed so pervasive that Congress held hearings on the issue in 1990. Both the FDA and the American Medical Association (AMA) published policy statements regarding physicians' acceptance of gifts and gave the FDA power to intercede if it deemed it necessary. But it appears that the pharmaceutical industry's ability to influence the public just keeps growing.

In 1997, the FDA decided to permit pharmaceutical companies to advertise various drugs on TV and radio. Because air time is very expensive, these spots will be too short to permit the listing of possible side effects. Many believe that this kind of advertising is irresponsible. In addition, physicians fear that patients will demand drugs without understanding their consequences. Managed care shares the trap of socialized medicine, in which it is easier to give into the patients' demands than risk their rejection.

The medical journal *Biological Psychiatry* featured an editorial saying that the health care industry emphasizes therapeutic drugs "at the expense of other modalities: psychotherapy, social approaches; nutritional, herbal, and natural remedies; rehabilitation, general hygienic measures, nonpatentable drugs, or other alternative approaches." There are many who feel this way, but they remain voices in the wilderness.

The authors are not knocking the pharmaceutical industry, which has, in fact, made many meritorious contributions to health care. The reader should bear in mind that the dietary supplement industry, while apparently at loggerheads with the pharmaceutical industry, has learned its marketing tricks from multinational drug firms. Many manufacturers or distributors of dietary supplements have made "hyped" comments about the their products' health benefits, making the purveyance of "crap in a can" not uncommon. Remember, the halls of both conventional and alternative health care are far from perfect. Pots often call kettles black.

The New Medicine

Whether the FDA is actually ensuring the safety of the drugs and medical devices we use, new products and techniques are changing our world. Prosthetic devices permit disabled people to live rich, full lives. Organ transplants — particularly kidney transplants — are performed on a daily basis. Children once destined to be midgets take growth hormones that will assure normal stature. The future looks even brighter because of the good work of regulatory agencies and medical innovations.

Several American companies are working furiously to create substitutes for human blood. Soon trauma victims will be transfused with blood replacements on the spot with no need for typing of blood. All risk from contaminated blood will disappear because the transfused material was never inside a human body. Blood shortages will be eliminated, and the synthetic substitutes will have an indefinite shelf life.

Work on spinal cord injuries is progressing beyond anyone's most fervent expectations. The possibility of regenerating the damaged nerves no longer falls into the realm of science fiction. In fact, the possibility of regenerating any severely injured body part looms on the horizon. With progress in cloning, the replacement of body parts is neither a dream nor a nightmare, but an eventuality we must address.

Nevertheless, the road of scientific discovery doesn't always lead to the betterment of mankind. Sometimes research falls into potholes created by politics, finances, or licensing agreements. One pothole swallowed hopes for a new, speedy way to determine HIV levels in blood. A nucleic acid analyzing machine called TaqMan is currently fighting its way out of that hole.

Roche Molecular Systems holds the patent on the analytic technique on which TaqMan is based. To use the technique, scientists need short pieces of nucleic acids. Roche's licensing agreement with a subsidiary of Perkin-Elmer prevents the firm from making or marketing these acids to be used diagnostically. If a researcher uses TaqMan as a diagnostic tool for measuring HIV levels in patients' blood rather than as a research tool, he violates a licensing agreement. Thus, business interests can supersede public health concerns.

This situation is most troubling considering that viral load measurements are crucial to AIDS treatment, for these serve as markers of both health status and the effect of therapy. At the time of this writing, Roche's assay is currently the only one available for quantifying HIV that has FDA approval.

While Roche is concerned that the equipment too easily generates a false positive, others believe that accuracy would be improved if the equipment were used more widely. Use by both industrial researchers and academics could yield effective new ideas for overcoming the problem. Roche may also be concerned that competitors who have free use of the system will gain an advantage in the marketplace, so the territory of proprietary technology is jealously guarded.

Meanwhile, a potentially lifesaving cancer treatment is mired in patent controversy. Johns Hopkins researchers hold patents on methods and materials involved in isolating large quantities of cells that can generate healthy blood cells and replenish the immune system. Called stem cells, these undifferentiated cells divide and produce a mature, fully functional cell. A machine exists that can be used to concentrate a patient's stem cells and regenerate his or her immune system following radiation and chemotherapy. The courts are now trying to decide whether the company that manufacturers the machine infringed on the university's patents.

All around the world, researchers involved in the Human Genome Project are attempting to determine the complete human genetic code. Researchers at Stanford University developed a machine that can inexpensively make substances critical to this project. One company received an exclusive license from Stanford to market the substance to researchers but not to sell the machine itself. Some scientists believe that Stanford's action is "counterproductive to the goal of completing the Human Genome Project as quickly as possible."

Cases such as these three raise difficult questions about intellectual property, technology, and the need to move science forward quickly. Although many researchers are motivated by the thirst for knowledge and the excitement of discovery, man cannot live on knowledge alone. There must be a roof over his head and shoes on his feet.

As government funding becomes increasingly difficult to come by, research scientists have to be more creative about funding. Licensing agreements with pharmaceutical and engineering giants certainly do infuse funds, which keep basic science going. At the other end of the road, when a discovery is made, licensing agreements may slow the transfer of the "property" to the public.

Conclusion

Even as we reap the vast benefits of medical technology, ethical dilemmas constantly confront us: Will the innovations be available to everyone equally? Will poor people be entitled to the same techniques as the rich? Who will pay for poor people's procedures? Who will make the decisions? In most of the world — in undeveloped countries as well as in America's inner cities and rural areas — access to the miracles of modern medicine is sometimes nonexistent. Maybe these impediments to the availability of modern technology will fuel even more interest in the exploration of natural remedies such as botanicals and herbs.

Meanwhile, those who can partake of the veritable font of medical miracles are questioning modern medicine's apparent failures. There is no doubt that people who enjoy the benefits of modern Western medicine live longer and are healthier than those in any other system of healing.

Still, cancer rates for American citizens are higher than for any other nationality. Throughout the Western world, the common cold still lays us low. Arthritis still cripples scores of adults and children. AIDS, cancer, and heart disease continue to kill thousands each year, and, in many cases, treatments are as debilitating as the disease. Radiation therapy can damage coronary arteries, increasing the risk of heart disease. Chemotherapy robs vitality and impairs the immune system. Surgery involves risks, expense, and sometimes long recuperation. Confronted by such issues, Americans are taking a long, hard look at conventional medicine. Apparently, we do not always like the answers.

3

Conventional Medicine Wars
With Alternative Medicine

Inequities in the delivery of health care services; escalating costs of medical care, medicines, and insurance; ills for which there are no cures; and injuries resulting from the use of conventional drugs and treatment are the problems that beset conventional or allopathic medicine. Because Americans are increasingly troubled by these issues, and are often dissatisfied by the health care they have been receiving, they have been seeking alternatives.

According to research conducted by Harvard Medical School in 1992, two-thirds of Americans use alternative health care. The statistics show that homeopathy is the most popular alternative among baby boomers, and dietary supplements are most popular among older Americans. Another survey indicated that 34 percent of patients had used at least one unconventional therapy — that's 61 million Americans. No doubt, many of these people were glued to the PBS production *Healing and the Mind,* which attained twice the ratings usually achieved by PBS at that time of year. Hosted by Bill Moyers, the show looked at the mind's power to cure. In 1993, *Newsweek* reported that almost half of all medical schools now offer at least some instruction in mind-body interaction.

Anyone who watches TV or reads a newspaper is certain to have heard about alternative medicines. One widely publicized story involves the wife of *Penthouse* publisher Bob Guccione. When she was told that she had stage-four breast cancer, Mrs. Guccione refused chemotherapy, which she regarded as "poison," and turned to an alternative — hydrazine sulfate. Two years later, she appeared on television looking healthy and swearing her tumors had disappeared.

In Texas, Stanislaw Burzynski, M.D., deals in an alternative called antineoplastons. This anticancer therapy has brought him close scrutiny

44

by the FDA and the Texas state medical board. In 1996, he was tried for insurance and mail fraud. Despite the contention of the trial, Dr. Burzynski reportedly earned $12 million that year. Thus, any press may be good press. Recently, Dr. Burzynski was exonerated in a trial that left the alternative medical community even more embittered about regulatory agencies' attitudes toward their profession.

Essiac, an herbal preparation that is purported to cure cancer, was formulated by a Canadian nurse in the 1920s. Its popularity never diminishes, yet the allopathic community rejects it as "ineffective." Interestingly, some alternative medical practitioners reject it as well.

Increasing interest in alternative medicine can be seen as a circular path. As Americans became interested in alternative medicine, the media began to feature people and products involved in the field. When the media focused on a particular alternative, people began to seek it out. In recent years, a media blitz about the powers of natural substances such as melatonin and garlic has generated increased demand for these products. In addition, manufacturers, entrepreneurs, and promoters began to see alternative medicine as a lucrative field. More and more products and services became available. As money was poured into advertising, the fires of alternative medicine burned brightly. Eventually, given the nature of the open market, some entrepreneurs began to offer inferior products, and some practitioners made bogus claims about therapies in an attempt to make a quick and easy buck. In an effort to get to the truth, the Office of Alternative Medicine (OAM) was initiated through Congressional mandate in 1992. OAM's task is to ensure that alternatives receive adequate scientific investigation. The agency is charged with identifying the alternative medicine community and issues of concern to it. In addition, one if its first tasks was to establish a research agenda. Grants were to be awarded, and the agency would conduct site visits to "seek out and evaluate new opportunities for medical therapy."

Unfortunately, the OAM has no power to deal with transgressions, but it can make informal recommendations to regulatory agencies. Funded through the National Institutes of health, the agency has an annual operating budget of $7.48 million dollars, less than the quarterly advertising budget that a multinational pharmaceutical company will spend to promote a single product.

Among the first alternative practices studied were nonpharmacologic treatments of PMS, the use of antineoplastons on brain tumors, and the evaluation of imagery — also known as visualization — and psychotherapy as treatments for patients with adenoid cystic carcinoma. The agency also conducted or participated in various workshops. One dealt with ethnobotany, the use of natural products in the practice of folk medicine. Another discussed the application of traditional Native American approaches and treatments to allopathic medicine.

Almost from the beginning, the Office of Alternative Medicine ran into difficulties. Its first director was considered far too conservative and did not stay in office very long. Wayne B. Jonas, M.D., a former lieutenant colonel in the army, became the second director. Dr. Jonas defines alternative medicine as "those practices used for the prevention and treatment of disease that are not taught widely in medical schools, nor generally available in hospitals." Although courses on alternative medicine are now being offered in approximately thirty medical schools, Dr. Jonas points out that use of nonconventional treatments is frequently rebuffed by the medical establishment. He claims, nonetheless, that more than 50 percent of American doctors practice or recommend an unconventional therapy to their patients. One frequently recommended alternative is nutritionally oriented chiropractic medicine.

Alternatives to Traditional Physicians

Long shunned by physicians, chiropractic practitioners filed an antitrust lawsuit against the American Medical Association (AMA) in 1976. In 1990, the U.S. Court of Appeals upheld a district court decision that had found the AMA guilty of an unlawful boycott against chiropractors. Now, more than twenty-five million Americans — many of whom are referred by physicians — regularly seek the services of a chiropractor. Practitioners of chiropractic medicine believe that misalignments of the vertebrae of the spine can produce a host of symptoms, many of which can be eliminated by correcting the alignment. Millions of Americans now swear that chiropractic manipulation successfully treats such complaints as stiffness or pain in the back and legs. Their faith that chiropractic medicine has far-reaching health consequences and can be used to treat and prevent other illnesses is growing.

Chiropractors are not the only alternative physicians who have gained foothold in America. Many Americans visit Oriental medical doctors (O.M.D.s). These health care practitioners do not actually hold a doctorate, but they may complete a four-year master's program in Oriental medicine. The knowledge base they acquire can be more varied and complete than the knowledge imparted in some medical schools. O.M.D.s are usually not permitted to prescribe drugs or perform surgery. They may, however, be associated with and direct the prescribing of licensed physicians.

Naturopathic doctors (N.D.s) practice holistic health care. Three accredited naturopathic medical schools in America train such physicians for four years following their receipt of an undergraduate degree. Approximately a dozen states now license naturopathic doctors, and in some of these, N.D.s can prescribe drugs and perform minor surgery.

Naturopaths provide botanical medicine, manipulation, and homeopathy. The latter, as you may know, is one of the most popular forms of alternative medicine today. Formulated by the German physician Samuel Hahnemann in the late 1700s, homeopathy uses minute doses of particular substances, often botanical in origin, to stimulate the body's natural defenses against disease. Instead of focusing on causes, homeopaths focus on symptoms as experienced by the patient, because they believe that each person is unique and experiences a disease differently.

Two or three decades ago, osteopathic medicine was considered a branch of alternative medicine. In recent times, the margins between conventional M.D.s and osteopaths have eroded. Today, osteopaths (D.O.s) are trained in medical schools that are the equivalent of those in which students receive M.D.s. Osteopathic doctors go through internships and residencies and take equivalent medical boards. Many residency training programs and specialty fellowship programs include both medical and osteopathic school graduates. D.O.s are licensed to diagnose and treat all medical conditions and to prescribe drugs. The major difference between the two is that D.O.s can practice manipulative therapy. Nevertheless, a number of D.O.s turn their backs on osteopathic concepts and practice allopathic medicine.

Osteopathic students actually spend more than 150 hours in classrooms and clinics learning the unique principles of osteopathy. The key phrase here is neuromuscular skeletal system — the interactions between nerves, muscles, and bones. Osteopaths practice allopathic medicine with special attention to the neuromuscular skeletal system.

Their medical approach includes — but is not limited to — correcting imbalances, injuries, or tensions in the system. Osteopaths use manipulative therapy as an adjunct to other modalities, such as surgery and chemotherapy.

If, for instance, an osteopath is treating a patient who has an infectious disease, the practioner might use manipulation as an adjunct to promoting movement of bodily fluids. Manipulation can, for example, promote good blood circulation or increase lymph movement through the lymph nodes. Lymph is a liquid that carries the antigens that help the body form antibodies. When an antigen is exposed to the immune cells circulating in the lymph nodes, the development of antibodies increases. By manipulating various muscles and fibrous membranes, the practitioner believes he can relax restricted motion and increase lymph flow. Osteopaths believe in these techniques; allopathic physicians most often consider them to be hogwash.

The Sum Is Greater Than the Parts

Generally speaking, the public today has embraced a more holistic approach to health. The modern holistic approach emphasizes a combination of exercise, emotional balance, and proper diet. In simple terms, a holistic approach means a move towards a healthy lifestyle.

People have become increasingly aware of the role that stress plays in poor health. Heart disease, hypertension, stroke, and body aches have all been associated with excess tension. Americans today know that only they can effect the lifestyle changes necessary to improve their health; in fact, 90 percent of Americans say that they have responsibility for their own health. Many of these people seek to improve their health through diet; they try to lose weight and seek to avoid fats, caffeine, and salt. More than 65 percent of Americans say they would rather cure an illness by changing their diet than by taking medicine. The evidence suggests that only a few people actually make the necessary lifestyle changes, but this core of health-conscious individuals is increasing.

Adherents of holistic medicine are apt to consider the effects that the mind has on the body. Millions eagerly snatch up copies of self-help books, such as Deepak Chopra's *Ageless Body, Timeless Mind,* and turn to such alternatives as visualization to help them combat disease. Herbert Benson,

M.D., head of Harvard's Mind/Body Institute, says that people have become "dissatisfied with routine medicine that's strictly drugs and surgery." The mind-body connection is a prevalent concept in most ancient medical systems. Although perceived as "innovative" these days, the concepts are really very old.

In a poll conducted in 1996 by Time/CNN, 82 percent of the respondents said they believed in the healing power of personal prayer, and in a survey of 269 physicians, 99 percent said they believed religious convictions can contribute to healing. So many people believe in the mind's influence on health that mind/body institutes have been established at prestigious medical centers in Ohio, New Jersey, and Tennessee. Dr. Andrew Weil has captured the public's attention with his concepts of self-healing for the body.

In Europe, people are heavy consumers of complementary medicine. In Germany, homeopathic medicine is practiced widely, and doctors may prescribe the herbal medication valerian for mild cases of anxiety. In Britain, there are more than thirty thousand practitioners of complementary medicine, and packaged herbal remedies are sold alongside drugs in many stores. In these countries, the cost-effectiveness of alternative medicine is becoming increasingly apparent. Some health maintenance organizations (HMOs) in the United States have integrated alternative medical strategies and have seen a lowering of overall costs as well as indications that patients are quite healthy and sometimes even more satisfied.

In August 1997, Daniel Freeman Marina Hospital in the Los Angeles area began a program that permitted the practice of acupuncture under the supervision of a licensed acupuncturist from Emperor's College of Traditional Oriental Medicine in Santa Monica. The following month, Los Angeles's Cedars-Sinai Medical Center announced it was beginning a complementary medicine program that will offer acupuncture, herbal medicine, massage therapy, homeopathy, and chiropractic. A New York newspaper called this "one of the most convincing signs that alternative health is moving into the mainstream."

Alternatives to Synthetic Drugs

We have seen that homeopathy is one of the most popular forms of alternative or complementary medicine. According to industry surveys, homeopathic remedies and herbal supplements are showing the strongest market growth among natural products.

More than twenty-eight million Americans are currently using herbal supplements. In 1991, they spent $445 million on them; by 1995, spending had increased to $772 million; by the end of 1996, sales of herbal products had reached $2 billion. Oxford Health Plans, a large managed health care company, includes some herbal-based products in its mail order vitamin catalog. Apparently, company administrators believe that the use of supplements can lead to lower health care costs. The economic reality is that herbal remedies cost half that of prescription remedies.

To address this increasing interest, health care givers, scientists, and members of the dietary supplement industry met in Washington, D.C., in October 1996 to discuss the early stage of developing a natural formulary. They recognize the need for authoritative standards and information sources on natural remedies. Uncertainty about the safety and efficacy of dietary supplement products prevails, despite the fact that alternative health care strategies are being used increasingly as first-line therapy by many individuals worldwide.

As the emphasis in medicine has shifted to prevention, people have realized that they can use herbs as "tonics" to promote good health instead of using drugs to cure disease. Herbs are now being used to improve circulation, prevent cancer, and enhance immune function. In addition, herbs are often perceived to have health benefits because of their long-term use in traditional or ethnic medical disciplines.

Herbal remedies and botanical extracts are now being increasingly used in the formulation of dietary supplements, and allopathic physicians are discovering the merits of these nutriceuticals. According to Andrew Weil, M.D., head of the Program in Integrative Medicine at the University of Arizona Medical School in Tucson, "Herbs may take longer to work, and the effects may be less dramatic at the outset, but they can be just as potent as conventional drugs."

Many people believe that natural substances are kinder to the human body. Richard Podell, M.D., M.P.H., is a clinical professor of family medicine at Robert Wood Johnson Medical School in New Jersey. He says, "I have a group of patients who've had bad side effects with drugs, and for these people, herbs become very attractive."

Mitchell Gaynor, M.D., director of medical oncology at Strang Cancer

Prevention Center in Manhattan, recommends several herbal formulas as part of the total treatment for cancer. Dr. Gaynor says, "This is no longer fad or folklore." These are signs that herbal medicine is here to stay.

Many clinicians, however, are reluctant to accept the accounts in traditional writings of herbals' or botanicals' therapeutic effects. Some scientists have referred to the Dietary Supplement Health Education Act of 1994 as the prime example of a mechanism to promote consumer fraud in recent years. At the other extreme are advocates of herbal medicine who believe that herbs can do no wrong. These people are apt to forget that some of the most toxic agents known to humankind — deadly nightshade, hemlock, avenging angel — are of plant origin. Herbal experts generally agree that children and pregnant or nursing women shouldn't use herbs except under a doctor's supervision.

Julian Whitaker, M.D., says that natural remedies are often overlooked by conventional physicians because "there is little money to be made in the use of natural remedies, regardless of how beneficial they may be for the patient." He points out that in a single year, sales for one or two major prescription drugs surpass revenues for the entire nutritional supplement industry.

In discussing herbal medicines or any alternatives, the medical and scientific establishment sometimes relies on catchphrases to put them down. Wallace Sampson, M.D., clinical professor of medicine at Stanford University School of Medicine, has compared the alternative medicine movement to the myth of the solitary hero against the world. Proponents of alternative medicine frequently — perhaps too frequently — see themselves as the underdog brought to heel by bigger, more powerful, richer establishment fixtures. They claim that their inexpensive and revolutionary treatments are deliberately sabotaged because they would detract from the conventional money-makers: chemotherapy, radiation, and surgery.

As writer John Sedgwick put it in the August 1997 issue of *Self,* "Somehow, medical science's very opposition is seen as proof that the unconventional remedy works." This mind-set is dangerous because it permits unscrupulous quacks to operate with increasing ease.

Sedgwick's article, which details cases of "junk medicine," leans heavily on twists of phrase to make his point. He says, for instance, that people from the establishment call acupuncture a version of transcutaneous electrical nerve stimulation "which has long been recognized in the West as a pain blocker." If acupuncture is a "version" of an accepted painblocker, then it, too, is beneficial.

Sedgwick also claims that proponents of alternatives tout the "beneficence of Mother Nature as opposed to the supposed evils of modern chemistry." He does not, however, go on to discuss the possibility of recognizing the former without adhering to the latter. Then he quotes a scientist who points out that what is important about a remedy is not whether it is alternative or conventional, but whether it is proven safe and efficacious through the "time-honored" scientific method. He also says, "Another common strategy is to tout an alternative's origins in the long ago and far away, as if anything that is of the here and now couldn't possibly be any good." Why is it acceptable to laud time in defense of the establishment but not in the defense of alternatives?

The bottom line questions remain: Does the medicine work? Is it safe? The difficulty can be keeping an open mind long enough to prove or disprove the efficacy of a technique or substance. One must be willing to cast out old methods — no matter how time-honored they may be — if newer ones prove better. No one — alternative or establishment — thinks we should go back to drilling holes in people's heads to let out the evil spirits that cause disease.

Modern physicians should be preoccupied with "what works" regardless of the origin of an intervention, be it alternative or conventional. The terms "alternative" and "conventional" foster a dichotomy of medicine that is destructive. Furthermore, jargon such as "integrated health care" does not help because it acknowledges the dichotomy. The age of pluralistic medicine is upon us, and any medical intervention that is effective and safe should be applied.

Seeking Scientific Evidence

As controversy about the use of herbs increases, more emphasis is being placed on scientific identification of the potential therapeutic value and safety of herbal remedies. Today, many American universities train pharmacognosists, pharmacists who specialize in plant medicine. In 1996, the American Chemical Society (ACS) entered into an agreement with the American Society of Pharmacognosy to publish the *Journal of Natural*

Products. Founded in 1876, the ACS is a not-for-profit membership organization that is now the largest scientific society in the world. It is considered a world leader in fostering scientific education and research, as well as the public's understanding of science. With the *Journal of Natural Products*, the ACS brings the public original research that applies fundamental chemical and biological principles to the study of natural products.

Although the ACS is a world leader, the society may have few powers of advocacy. Recommendations for action are often ignored, and the approach to herbal medicine in the United States is retarded in comparison to many European countries.

Herbalism may be the oldest and most common healing technique. Fossilized evidence in Switzerland indicates that as long ago as 4000 B.C., humans were extracting opium from the opium poppy (*Papaver somniferum*) and using it to relieve pain. Asians, Africans, South Americans, and even Europeans have been using herbal-based medicines since time immemorial.

Five thousand years ago, the Sumerians were using caraway and thyme for healing. In ancient Egypt, onions and garlic were used as remedies for a multitude of conditions. In ancient Greece, a plant called silphion was so valuable that it was worth its weight in silver. This plant, which seems to have been a species of *Ferula* (giant fennel), may have been an effective oral contraceptive. In 2800 B.C., one Chinese herbalist listed 366 plant drugs in the *Pen Ts'ao*. Ancient treatment philosophies such as the Ayurvedic medicine of India and traditional Chinese medicine use herbal products as part of a complete health care system involving mind-body medicine and other natural options.

The role of herbs in conventional Western medicine is not new. In 360 B.C., Hippocrates, the Greek known as the Father of Physicians, recorded upwards of three hundred plant remedies. The Greek physician Pedanius Dioscorides (c. 40-c. 90 A.D.) recommended that a particular species of crocus be soaked in wine and made into a poultice for the treatment of tumors. We know now that the plant is a member of the lily family and contains colchicine, an alkaloid that is currently used in the production of a treatment for granulocytic leukemia.

Until the eighteenth century, physicians prepared and dispensed medications that were more often than not picked from their own gardens.

Prior to World War II, herbal medications were listed in the *U.S. Pharmacopoeia (USP)*, the official listing of accepted medicines. Obviously, herbal medicines did not fall out of favor overnight.

Herbs in History

Between 1470 and 1670, hundreds of herbals — botanical books with illustrations of herbs and descriptions of their useful properties — were written. Particularly popular in England and Germany, the herbals contained meticulously executed illustrations and text detailing the uses, harvesting, and preparation of the various "drugs." Intermingled with the accurate information in the herbals, however, were many descriptions of the magical powers of plants. In many cases, these powers were based on the doctrine of signatures.

One of the earliest therapeutic systems, the doctrine of signatures claimed that Providence provides remedies at the place where the disease originates or among the victims themselves. Subscribers to the doctrine also believed that God had marked all things that had therapeutic benefit and had left signs indicating the uses of natural objects. An herb resembling a specific human organ or part would, therefore, be effective in treating that organ. A heart-shaped leaf was thought to be useful in the treatment of heart ailments, and a kidney-shaped leaf was thought effective for kidney troubles. Ginseng root's resemblance to the human body is believed to be one of the reasons for its early application in the treatment of many body ailments.

The doctrine of signatures may have played a large part in sounding the death knell for herbal medicine. Although superstition and magic have no role in medicine, we may, in some cases, have thrown the baby out with the bath water. The story of Philippus Aureolus Theophrastus Bombastus Von Hohenheim, known as Paracelsus, is a case in point.

Letting the Negative Outweigh the Positive

A Swiss physician and alchemist who came to prominence in the early 1500s, Paracelsus is considered "Perhaps the greatest reformer of Renaissance medicine" by medical historian Dr. Benjamin Gordon. He has, nonetheless, been almost universally forgotten by the medical establishment. In reviewing Paracelsus's life, one may get the impression that he could not resolve his own scientific beliefs. Quite the contrary. Paracelsus was consistent in his message, a message that upset his peers and prompted his travels throughout Europe. He was scorned and hounded by members of his profession, a phenomenon that continues today with some alternative, or lateral thinking, physicians. The scorned physician comes in two distinct types: one that deserves the rejection, and one that has a lot to offer. Middle ground does not exist for such an individual.

One of the first advocates of chemical remedies, Paracelsus is recognized by *Dorland's Illustrated Medical Dictionary* as the man whose research led to the use of lead, sulfur, iron, and arsenic in pharmaceutical chemistry. He may have been the first to discover ether, and he introduced and named laudanum, a tincture of opium still used today. Cited as being far ahead of his time in many of his observations — including those on metabolic and occupational diseases — he was the first to say that coitus was a cause of gonorrhea.

Paracelsus had daily contact with his patients, among whom were numerous laborers and other common people. His genius came from his use of what he learned in daily clinical contact rather than in books. In Paracelsus' own words, "The human mind knows...[what] his eyes see and his hands touch, that is his teacher." Powerful words for modern medicine in which talking to patients or conducting a clinical examination has been replaced by high technology.

Contrary to the custom of his times, which often measured a surgeon's reputation by the amount of blood on his clothing, Paracelsus believed in the necessity of clean surgery. He said, "I have often seen the ignorance of you surgeons, while the wounds fairly stank and poured forth a foul pus." It is no surprise that Paracelsus had few friends in his chosen profession of healing.

Paracelsus believed that nature was the proper and best physician. If, however, nature refused to cooperate, then the "external physician" must support the "internal physician." He advised physicians "to use alchemy" — the forerunner of the science of chemistry — in preparing herbal medicines. Most moderns associate the study of alchemy with attempts to turn lead into gold. Although this endeavor certainly did occur, alchemy is actually a philosophical and medical tradition. The underlying idea is that a substance's energies can be purified so that they may be manipulated to create an enhanced physical substance — be it an herbal remedy or gold. It is a system of physical transmutation that was central to much of the scientific research in all ancient civilizations. Alchemists prepared extracts and formulas, particularly tinctures and essences. In fact, alchemists developed many of the techniques still used for processing plants and volatile oils.

According to Paracelsus, obtaining a "perfect medicine" required separating the pure from the impure. He reminded practitioners that God did not give us the medicines already prepared: "He wants us to cook them ourselves." He also said that all things are toxic if they are not taken with regard to proper dosage.

Unfortunately, Paracelsus's practical ideas about medicine were ignored, despite his tremendous success in curing or alleviating conditions when all other physicians had failed. Not only was he superstitious, he had no medical degree. Furthermore, his pharmaceutical system was not in keeping with the commerce of the apothecaries whose drugs he did not use. A egotist of the first order, Paracelsus also had a violent temper that was fueled by the jealousy and hatred of his colleagues. Accused of poisoning people with his use of metals like antimony, no wonder he frequently "skipped town." Paracelsus may have been murdered by hirelings of either the physicians or apothecaries.

Though he may have been a mystic, though he depended on herbs and often on superstition, Paracelsus was probably the first physician to practice empiric medicine at the scientific level. Eventually, scientific medicine became the order of the day. People began to reject the doctrine of signatures and stopped turning to their gardens for medicines; instead, they headed to the apothecary shops. If the apothecaries had exercised more tolerance towards Paracelsus, they would have been more successful. Perhaps there is a hidden message here for managed care organizations and health care institutions that have been slow to delve into the increasingly popular art of complementary medicine.

Pharmacist and Physician Feud

In seventeenth-century France, a running battle occurred between apothecaries and physicians. All the doctors of the era believed that purging and bleeding could cure the vast majority of ailments. King Louis

XIV, however, loathed being bled and flatly refused the procedure. He did, however, submit to purges (an increasingly popular practice today).

At this time in history, a particularly prominent physician was Gui Patin (1602–72). Twice dean of the Paris medical school, Patin believed that medical education should center around the reading of Hippocrates, Galen, and Aristotle. He scoffed at the Arabs, whose contribution to medicine consisted of nothing but the enriching of apothecaries, with medicinal formulas consisting of "sugared and honeyed alteratives... We save more sick people with a good lancet and a pound of senna than the Arabians can with their syrups and opiates."

Apparently, Patin's medical beliefs were popular. He amassed quite a fortune, as evidenced by his large house in Paris and his country estate complete with a huge library and famous wine cellar.

In seventeenth-century France, however, physicians were apt to prescribe any number of elaborate compositions. Human afterbirth was used to cure pimples; essence of human urine was often used to cure the vapors, the seventeenth-century equivalent of depression; and compositions could consist of entire animals, scrappings from the skulls of dead men, or animal excrement (white peacock's dung was favored for epilepsy). The formula might be as complex as Eau de Vie de Dresde, which had 118 ingredients.

Patin preferred to follow a more simple route. His favorite medicinal was senna; he simply ignored the fact that it had reached France via the Arabs. He also used laxative syrups of cassia, rhubarb, or prune juice. Patin and the French became obsessed with bowel function, an obsession that still exists in many European countries. Bear in mind, great leaders of this century acknowledged digestive function as the key to health. Winston Churchill is alleged to have characterized the two greatest pleasures in life to be swallowing and defecating. Perhaps good digestive function is one of the few historic examples of agreement between the French and the English.

The apothecaries and the faculty of the medical school in Paris had been in a power struggle for as long as anyone could remember. The physicians wanted to be in charge and the apothecaries wanted to be independent with the right to practice medicine themselves. The faculty of the medical school published manuals showing people how to make their own medicines. Patin, who seemed at least as eager to harm the apothecaries as to help his patients, believed the manuals "ruined the apothecaries of Paris."

In London, the physicians struck a truce with the apothecaries. Physicians permitted them to establish an independent company in exchange for their agreement to accept the supervision of the medical school faculty. In 1700, there were about one hundred thirty trained physicians serving a population of seven hundred thousand Londoners. Obviously, the scarcity of doctors ensured good fees for those who practiced medicine. A physician could expect to earn from 2,000 to 3,000 pounds a year (equivalent to roughly $4,000 to $6,000 a year, which was a fortune then). Queen Anne's physician actually left an estate valued at one million pounds sterling ($1.7 million).

The common people could not normally afford a physician's fees, so apothecaries picked up many of these patients. An apothecary's bills for an illness were less than those of a physician but still hefty. These shopkeepers were prohibited from charging for advice; they could only profit from what they sold — and profit they did, gaining a fair reputation along the way.

So conciliatory was the alliance between London's physicians and apothecaries that the Worshipful Society of Apothecaries of London has retained the right to issue medical qualifications equivalent to degrees in medicine. In addition, these apothecaries retained other rights in common law, such as the right to herd goats across the bridges of the River Thames in London.

By the early nineteenth century, a new science of pharmacognosy was emerging. This study deals with the biological, biochemical, and economic features of natural drugs and their constituents — drugs whose origins are in the plant and animal kingdom. The word, coined in 1815 by C. A. Seydler, a medical student in Germany, is drawn from the Greek *pharmakon*, meaning "drug" and *gnosis*, meaning "knowledge." Pharmacognosy is considered the earliest discipline of pharmaceutical education.

Synthetic Drugs Take Over

In the mid-nineteenth century, pharmacology — the study of the changes produced in people and animals through the use of chemical substances — entered the world of medicine. The Philadelphia College of Pharmacy and

Science, the first pharmaceutical school in the United States, was established in 1821, and the American Pharmaceutical Association was formed in 1851. European universities had established the programs about fifty years earlier. The most notable source of modern therapeutics was the University of Edinburgh in Scotland.

Due to the establishment of these groups, we were standing at the doorway of a new era: Chemotherapy would now rule. Researchers began to conduct animal experiments using isolated and purified active substances in the pursuit of ever-better drugs and the profit they would bring.

The constantly increasing size of the *United States Pharmacopoeia* — the legal standard for drugs since 1906 — bears witness to the growing number of prescription medications, but it does not attest to the number of medicines that are derived from a plant source. Digitalis, a commonly used heart medication, is derived from foxglove. The bark of the white willow tree provided the first analgesics, and today's aspirin pills are synthesized to duplicate the salicin found in its bark. The blood pressure medication Reserpine comes from an Asian shrub that has been used in India since ancient times. Quinine, derived from the bark of a tree, was the only drug available to treat malaria for three hundred years. It is still used today because the pathogen has become resistant to synthetic drugs. The ephedrine and pseudoephedrine used in many cold remedies are derived from the ephedra plant, which is known in traditional Chinese medicine as *ma huang.*

Thousands of children with leukemia have been saved through the use of vincristine and vinblastine, derived from the rosy periwinkle tree. Many of us are aware of taxol, a recently approved anticancer drug that is derived from a particular species of yew tree. In veterinary medicine, ivermectin, a fungal product, is widely used to kill internal worms in dogs, pigs, and horses. These are actually only a few examples of botanicals that can provide compounds of significant medicinal value.

It was not necessarily a lack of efficacy that caused the decline in herbal use; it was most often economics. With the Food and Drug Administration requiring extensive — and expensive — testing before a substance can be approved as a drug, the development of new drugs is not an undertaking suited for small businesses. Since natural substances cannot be patented, a company cannot recoup the expense of securing official drug status for an herb. However, when a synthetic drug is developed, a company has the exclusive right to market that product for as long as seventeen years, a right that, in some instances, can be extended to twenty-two years.

In the years since aspirin was first marketed, people in the Western world have perhaps become too used to taking a pill to cure what ails them. Perhaps we have been guilty of blindly accepting pharmaceuticals without questioning their cost, side effects, or possible alternatives. That is beginning to change.

Despite the widespread use of many synthetic drugs, we know relatively little about their long-term safety. In contrast, we have vast experience with many herbs and botanicals that have been part of the food chain for thousands of years. This does not mean that synthetic drugs are "bad," "unnatural," or "harmful."

Today's synthetic drugs are produced easily and economically. These drugs are often stronger, more consistent, and quicker-acting than their natural counterparts. Because pharmaceuticals are fast-acting, they can move people out of life-threatening situations. Few people would give a child herbal tea to cure a clinically diagnosed strep throat accompanied by a raging fever. Most of us know that an untreated strep throat can lead to heart problems. Untreated middle-ear infections (*otitis media*) can lead to hearing loss and delays in language development in children. In these cases, it is most prudent to give a child an antibiotic, stabilize his or her condition, and then, perhaps, use herbal remedies to augment the healing process. With less threatening conditions, however, it might be acceptable to use more natural remedies.

One might ask, "Why take sleeping pills or tranquilizers that can be habit-forming and leave you slow-witted if you can sip a cup of St. John's wort with the same soothing effects as the drugs?" Then, too, symptoms such as diarrhea, vomiting, and coughing are the body's way of eliminating toxins. If you completely suppress the symptoms, healing may take longer, but you don't have to suffer, either. Herbal remedies can sometimes ease discomfort without interrupting the healing process of the body.

Today, many Americans believe that there are herbal preparations that are as effective — possibly even more effective — than their synthetic counterparts. There is some evidence that microorganisms develop resistance to synthetic chemicals more readily than to plant-derived ones.

Plasmodium falciparum, a parasite that causes malaria, for instance, is resistant to synthetic drugs, while quinine, used since the 1600s, continues to be effective.

Another oft-cited example of the advantages of herbal medicine is saw palmetto (*Serenoa repens*). A small palm tree native to the West Indies and the southeast coast of the United States, the tree has berries that have traditionally been used to treat prostate conditions. A number of recent clinical studies were conducted using the fat soluble extract of the berries. Results reported in various medical journals indicate that the extract may be more effective in treating prostatic enlargement than synthetic drugs.

For example, the drug Proscar (Merck, Inc.) was shown in one study to be effective in less than 50 percent of those who had taken the drug for a full year. Extracts of the saw palmetto berries were shown to be effective in almost 90 percent of patients. In addition, Proscar has several negative side effects that are absent when the herbal remedy is used. For instance, saw palmetto users may not incur the decreased libido or impotence experienced by those who use Proscar. Another advantage of the herbal preparation is that it is only one quarter as expensive as the synthetic. Despite the fact that the FDA recognized saw palmetto's "statistically significant" effect, the agency refused to approve the herb for the treatment of enlarged prostrates. Known medically as benign prostate hyperplasia (BPH), this condition affects more than half of the men over the age of forty.

Conclusion

The marketing of synthetic products generates $100 billion in annual pharmaceutical industry revenues. No wonder many advocates of alternative medicine claim that natural alternatives are squelched in pursuit of greater profit. On the other hand, the medical establishment claims that advocates of alternative medicine are, at best, inferior scientists whose claims are not substantiated or, at worst, quacks and charlatans. Neither group appears particularly open-minded, and both, like Paracelsus and his critics, are too easily incited to angry words. Each camp has dug a moat around itself that cannot be crossed by parties from the other side. Now, however, an exciting new technology can provide a bridge between establishment medicine and advocates of herbal remedies.

4

Signal Transduction Technology

The lush foliage of the tropical rain forest in Arecibo, Puerto Rico, is interrupted by a large antenna. A satellite dish bigger than a football field, the structure listens for signals from outer space. When and if a signal — a transmitted or randomly received message — finally comes, a door to understanding the universe will open.

Meanwhile, amid the sterile white hubbub of the scientific laboratory lies a tiny oasis of silence. Under the microscope, investigators look within living cells for the signals or messages that initiate and control life on Earth. When they find them — as they do almost daily — the door to controlling disease opens a little wider.

The signals that swarm around us — whether from outer space or deep within our cells — can be the key to improving, or even continuing, life on Earth.

On a microscopic level, cells in the human body carry out their functions in response to signals or external stimuli. Within each cell, information is constantly being processed. A cell's hereditary information is coded in the form of DNA — deoxyribonucleic acid. DNA is constructed chemically from two long chains of building blocks twined together into a structure that is shaped like a double spiral or double helix. Portions of the DNA called genes are used as patterns from which RNA — ribonucleic acid — is formed. RNA consists of a single strand of chemical building blocks that are quite similar to the chemicals of the DNA strands. By reading the code in the RNA, the cell constructs proteins that are used to build the cell's structures and conduct chemical reactions. In brief, the cell functions by translating DNA to RNA to protein. The procedure involves numerous biochemical processes that occur when the cell is subjected to various stimuli.

Probably the most basic of the processes is the cell cycle. Molecular cycles in cells represent the most fundamental of biorhythms. Many writers have pointed to the advantages of recognizing the body's natural cycles in order to lead happier or more successful lives. Their books focus on gross cycles such as menstruation and the occurrence of major events such as menopause or andropause.

Biological rhythms are described in humans, animals, and plants. The individual who is credited with the popularization of biological rhythms is Dr. Wilhelm Fleiss, a German ear, nose, and throat physician who practiced in Berlin in the late nineteenth century and published a major work entitled *The Rhythm of Life: Foundations of an Exact Biology*. Many of his observations are focused on sexual theories or cycles.

Fleiss used his knowledge of cycles as a practical treatment device. He alleged that he had detected cyclical changes in the cells lining the nasal cavity and applied botanicals, such as cocaine, to treat emotional problems. Thus was born the practice of sniffing cocaine. Freud endorsed Fleiss's theories, characterizing them as major biopharmacological breakthroughs, perhaps in part to excuse his own cocaine addiction.

While we recognize macro-cycles of nature, or broad biological rhythms, only recently has attention been focused on rhythms at the cellular level. Very clear circadian rhythms such as cell division are well recognized. Furthermore, cell divisions in actively growing tissues show peaks of activity. It is known that the skin exhibits maximal rates of cell division during sleep. Thus, biological rhythms are synchronous with other rhythms, such as sleep, which occurs in darkness as the world turns and the moon, planets, and stars visably adopt a spatial relationship to Earth. Who said astrology is a worthless science?

Almost forty years ago, several scientists showed that cell division (mitosis) results from rhythms in the replication of basic nucleic acids: DNA and RNA. DNA and RNA are components of genetic programs, and the messages maintaining order occur during the cell cycle. Experiments at the University of Minnesota have shown that cancer cell division occurs in a rhythmic manner, with some variation in periodicity. It is known that signals are given to organelles (components within cells) in complex ways to undertake molecular activities. The process of signaling must presumably occur in a cyclical manner, and this cycle may be interrupted by external influences. The phenomenon of signal transduction, or the carrying of messages to cellular particles in order to "turn on" their functions, will be discussed in some detail. This concept is the basis of signal transduction technology.

The Cell Cycle

There are five distinct phases in the cell cycle:

G_0 is quiescence.

G_1, or Gap 1, is the time period between the division of the nucleus (mitosis) and the creation of new genetic material (DNA).

S-phase is the time period in which cellular DNA is replicated.

G_2 is the time period between completion of S-phase and the execution of mitosis.

M-phase (mitosis) is the stage in which the replicated DNA separates and a daughter cell forms.

When the cycle proceeds as it should, cells, tissues, and organs are healthy, but if any of the signals that control the process are interfered with, disease can develop. In recent years, cell biologists have made great strides in identifying the molecules that drive the cell cycle. We owe many of their discoveries to an innovation called signal transduction technology, which rests on the premise that information relating to control of the cell cycle is passed along various pathways.

To better understand this process, imagine that your TV screen is a human cell. To support the "life" on that screen — the life of a human cell — external signals must be passed along various pathways to the TV's electronic components. In a cell, signals are delivered through a biochemical process called signal transduction. The messages bring about a cascade of molecular and biochemical events that have diverse effects on cell functions. When something interferes with the molecules that control signal transduction, the communications mechanism within a cell is destroyed, and the cell will no longer function as it should.

Think about your TV again; if something interferes with your reception, there will be no picture on the screen. A television repairmen can then adjust the set's electrical components so that you will be able to see a picture. Scientists who understand the molecules involved in signal transduction may soon be able to "repair" a host of diseases.

Understanding cell signaling improves researchers' understanding of disease mechanisms and enables them to create new pharmaceuticals.

A New Era in Disease Treatment and Prevention

Cellular messengers come in a variety of forms. These messengers attach to a cell's surface, initiating events through a series of receptors and intermediate compounds that control cellular function. Perhaps the best known of the messengers are hormones — substances produced in one tissue that travel via the bloodstream to another tissue where they bring about such physiological activities as growth or metabolism. In addition, kinins, chains of amino acids, act locally to induce dilation of blood vessels and contraction of smooth or involuntary muscles, such as those in the intestinal walls. These and other messengers attach to cell membrane receptors, providing stimuli that affect cell processes, including proliferation and gene expression. The membrane receptors then pass the communications to secondary messengers — a complex array of enzymes and proteins.

Scientists now know that in all human cells, the cell cycle is governed by signal transduction pathways mediated by complexes of cyclin proteins, named for their cyclical appearance, and enzymes that are activated only when bound to a cyclin. These cyclin-dependent kinases — biochemical catalysts that render an enzyme active — are usually referred to as CDKs.

Twelve CDKs have thus far been identified, but studies have concentrated largely on what is called CDK-1, which plays a pivotal role in the control of cell division in plants and animals. In normal resting cells, CDK-1 is not expressed or is expressed at very low levels. Concentrations increase as the cell enters and passes through certain identified stages of replication. Several studies also suggest that CDK-1 functions in the initiation of mitosis — the process of cell division by which the nucleus divides. Cellular expression of CDK-1 is governed by exposure to cytokines, molecules of hormonelike protein and hormones. Cytokines affect physiological processes at a cellular level by inducing activity in cells. *Kinesis* means "movement" and *cyto* means "cells." When CDK-1 is expressed, a message is sent to a cell to initiate the events of cell division.

CDK-1 can be called the central information processing protein because its function involves the coordination of all events related to cell division. As the cell moves through the cell cycle, information concerning the activities of the cell is sent to CDK-1. As long as these signals indicate proper cell function, movement through the cycle continues. Evidence indicates that derangement in these signal processes may contribute to the development of a number of apparently unrelated diseases.

Several disease such as cancer, heart disease, AIDS, and viral infections have been associated with the overexpression and aberrant functioning of CDK-1. For example, the expression of this protein mediates the proliferation of vascular endothelial cells. These cells, from which capillaries sprout, line the circulatory system. Their proliferation is associated with the development of new blood vessels, a process known as angiogenesis. The development of new vessels is part of the process that leads to the development of diseases such as cancer, arthritis, and proliferative retinopathy of diabetes melitus. Angiogenesis also occurs during the process of wound healing and is, therefore, involved in the occlusion of arteries following certain heart operations.

Since the 1970s, scientists have known that angiogenesis is critical to the growth and metastasis of tumor cells. Blood vessels bring nourishment to these cells and carry away waste products. These blood vessels also provide a route by which cancerous cells can travel to different sites in the body, which is the process of metastasis.

Concrete evidence now supports a relationship between aberrant CDK-1 and cancer. Overexpression of the protein has been noted in 90 percent of the breast tumor cell lines examined, in all forty of the human cancer cells studied, and in all clinical gastric and colon carcinomas studied.

Through signal transduction technology, investigators have seen that CDK-4 targets the phosphorylation of the protein known as Rb. During phosphorylation, a phosphate group is added to the protein. Phosphorylation is one of many common chemical changes that occurs in molecules to make them more active. This chemical change plays a major role in many body processes, including signal transduction in cells. Researchers have noted that upon phosphorylation by CDKs, Rb loses its growth suppressive activity and permits the cell to enter its S-phase. Researchers at the Johns Hopkins Oncology Center and Howard Hughes Medical Institute have reported that phosphorylation at certain sites is critical to the development of some cancers including colorectal tumors.

Protein tyrosine phosphorylation is a physiological process critical to the regulation of cell growth. Two classes of enzymes act as switches, turning the process on or off. Anton M. Bennett, Ph.D., a postdoctoral fellow at Cold Spring Harbor Laboratory on Long Island, New York, has been attempting to better understand the enzymes' role in cellular functions. Dr. Bennett believes that this knowledge may contribute to the discovery of drugs that can control cancer and some neurological disorders. These drugs may well include naturally occurring substances such as herbs.

Scientists from the Harbor Branch Oceanographic Institution in Florida and Cornell University in New York have isolated a protein phosphatase inhibitor from a Caribbean sponge, *Dysidea etheria* de Laubenfels. Known as dysidiolide, the substance blocks an enzyme that acts as a catalyst in the cell cycle. By inhibiting mitosis, the compound is "potentially useful in the treatment of cancer," according to an item in *Chemical and Engineering News*.

Researchers' ability to interpret and modify cellular signals can help us to understand, prevent, and treat disease. Therefore, signal transduction technology will play an increasing role in uncovering new pharmaceuticals and in devising tests for the diagnosis of cancer and environmental carcinogens. Tests sensitive to the CDK-1 marker are now being used to detect the increased cell division often associated with chemically induced cancer in laboratory animals. Researchers can observe and measure the effects various substances have on cell signaling. They can screen compounds to identify those that are dangerous as well as those with promising therapeutic effects. In addition, signal transduction technology reveals novel pathways of action for potential drugs. As these previously undiscovered pathways are identified, they can be used in screening for other active compounds.

Novel Drugs Already Being Developed

A class of pharmaceuticals called antisense drugs has evolved because of scientists' increased knowledge of molecular signals. In designing antisense drugs, researchers must first identify a protein critical to the flourishing of a particular disease. The action of that protein is then blocked with a synthetic chemical that binds or glues itself to the messenger RNA that serves as the template for synthesis of the protein. Once the messenger is taken out of action, the protein cannot be synthesized.

Scientists hope to devise antisense drugs to which microorganisms cannot become resistant. These researchers are attempting to create tailor-made chunks of RNA that will get into the bacteria and bind to the RNA made by drug-resistant genes. Then the naturally occurring enzyme RNAase cuts up the combined RNA molecules, inactivating those genes responsible for drug resistance.

Several antisense drugs are currently in the testing stage. Lynx Pharmaceuticals of Hayward, California, in partnership with Schwarz Pharmaceuticals of Germany, is testing a drug targeted against a gene involved in regulation of the cell cycle. This drug is designed to prevent the buildup of scar tissue that occurs after surgical procedures, which will then open partially blocked arteries. Researchers are also studying the messenger RNA of the GAG gene, which is essential for replication of the AIDS virus. The substance currently being tested inhibits replication at several different stages in the cell cycle. Several other compounds being tested are anticancer drugs because they target the messenger RNA of protein kinase A, a cell-signaling molecule.

Unfortunately, there is no real way of predicting which part of the messenger RNA molecule will be accessible to bind with the drug. The drugs can, for instance, bind to blood-clotting factors. Some changes in clotting time have been noted during testing, but these changes appear to occur at doses higher than those needed to produce the positive effect. Another negative aspect of antisense drugs is their cost. During the initial research phase, it is costing approximately $1,000 to produce 1 gram of the drug. Market-scale production should lower the cost to between $50 to $100 per gram. Obviously, antisense drugs will not sell cheaply.

Other biochemical substances involved in cell signaling are being investigated as potential therapies. At the Whitehead Institute in Cambridge, Massachusetts, researchers have discovered a natural protein that may help combat tuberculosis. Called osteopontin because it was first seen in bone cells, this protein signals cells from the immune system, attracting them to the site of infection. Thanks to increased understanding of cell signals, researchers are also on the road to preventing one form of infertility.

Scientists at the University of Florida Brain Institute have found that males and females can become infertile when certain messenger molecules in the hypothalmus behave abnormally. "Mapping the site of these signaling mechanisms makes it a target for future drug therapies," says Satya Kalra, professor of neuroscience at the university's College of Medicine. Other diseases that may be affected by the control of molecular signals include cancer, AIDS, and some cardiovascular diseases.

Fulfilling the Promise of Nutriceuticals

At present, researchers are studying compounds contained in both synthetic and natural substances, such as herbal extracts. Approximately twenty companies worldwide are using signal transduction technology in the development of new drugs. They hope to isolate compounds that can then be submitted in a formal drug development route with standard regulatory pathways. However, signal transduction experiments with natural agents may lead to the development of dietary supplements that can be marketed without the extensive investigation required by the FDA or other regulatory agencies.

Signal transduction technology's role in the development of pharmaceuticals is particularly viable in the investigation of herbal and other natural medicines — the so-called nutriceuticals. The technology permits the identification of herbal extracts with low toxicity and positive therapeutic potential. In so doing, it eliminates many of the criticisms that had been leveled against natural medicines.

Proponents of natural medicinals have long been criticized for a lack of controlled studies. But double-blind controlled clinical trials are expensive and time-consuming. The dietary supplement industry does not have the financial resources, personnel, or facilities for conducting such trials. Multinational pharmaceutical companies are far more accustomed to conducting studies that must be filed with regulatory agencies.

Signal Transduction Technology at the
Heart of Dietary Supplement Development

Signal transduction technology now enables investigators to screen and investigate the effects of botanical extracts within molecular systems. The study of cell cycle protein expression also has the advantage of being an in vivo model. This means responses can be studied in organs and in the whole animal. Concrete evidence is obtained without the need for costly and time-consuming trials. The studies can also lead to increased understanding of the action of tumor suppressor proteins and carcinogenic pathways.

The dietary supplement industry may now run out of excuses when its platforms for the use of botanicals for health purposes are questioned. The industry can now seek the lower cost alternative of in vitro biotechnology methodology, such as signal transduction, to show the reputed benefits of dietary supplements. The Dietary Supplement Health and Education Act of 1994 permits statements about the effects of dietary supplements on body structure and function. What could be better than the use of in vitro studies involving signal transduction technology to support the wellness claims of herbals and other botanicals? This type of research may be the ideal pathway for screening botanicals for health applications.

Before signal transduction technology was developed, the efficacy of natural products was argued based on the weight of anecdotal evidence. Most members of the medical establishment and most scientific researchers scoffed at such evidence. Now, the precise chemical and biological activities (mechanisms of action) that produce desirable and predictable results can be identified. By using a combination of cellular and biochemical responses, researchers can identify extracts that affect targeted cell cycle proteins, have the capacity to enter the cell, and do not interact with nontarget proteins.

Treatments developed through signal transduction technology have the advantage of reaching the market more quickly and with less expense than products developed through traditional methods. In a single year, members of the Pharmaceutical Research and Manufacturers Association spend approximately $19 billion on research and development of new drugs for serious medical conditions. Industry members spent approximately $1.5 billion on the development of anticancer drugs in just one year. Of this amount, approximately 30 percent, or $450 million, was spent on synthesis, extraction, and screening.

Research and development costs in the pharmaceutical industry are high for many reasons. The FDA requires extensive toxicology studies before it will grant approval for a new drug. Conducting tests to assess safety includes disproving the possibility of carcinogenic potential, even for the offspring of drug users. These tests require repeated experimentation with animals. Signal transduction technology permits pharmacologists to look directly at a substance's effect on cells rather than wait until symptoms of toxicity develop in a test subject.

Signal transduction technology has found a particular role in defining the toxicological profile of many drugs, natural compounds, and environmental toxins. Monitoring the concentration of CDK-2 in rodents' serum, for instance, makes it possible to assess the carcinogenicity of a test chemical in ninety days, compared to the two years currently required. The observed outcomes can also be used to predict a compound's beneficial effects on cellular function. Dietary supplements that demonstrate therapeutic activity in vitro can then be available for sale, providing that the specific guidelines of the 1994 Dietary Supplement Health Education Act (see Appendix B) are followed. Some nutriceuticals will be grandfathered as dietary supplements, while other natural medicines and compounds can be marketed under the DSHEA without the need for investigational new drug applications to the FDA.

Currently, government guidelines do not permit dietary supplements to be used in the prevention or treatment of disease. Individuals are obviously very interested demonstrating health-giving benefits in order to support claims of body structure function. Such claims can then be permitted on the labels of dietary supplements. Signal transduction technology can, therefore, get efficacious therapies to the marketplace more quickly. The shortened time period means speedier access to needed drugs and lower costs for the consumer.

It is not surprising, then, that several companies in North America are studying the potential efficacy of botanical extracts. At one American company, researchers have been working with the National Cancer Institute's Laboratory of Tumor Cell Biology, screening traditional Chinese medicines for pharmacological agents. They are looking for herbs that have the ability to modulate the cell signaling pathways induced in certain HIV and cancer cell lines developed by the institute. The researchers hope to develop an understanding of various traditional herbs' effects on cell signaling pathways.

In the laboratory, investigators can identify substances in herbal extracts that have specific effects on cellular models. Once a positive response is noted, the historical use of the botanical that is the source of the extract is investigated, and further development of compounds with a history of toxicity or of poor bioavailability is then eliminated. A chemical within the extract is subsequently identified, and its mechanism of action is described.

Recent research has revealed a number of botanical extracts that do, indeed, affect the process of signal transduction. In some cases, herbal compounds have been shown to affect genes involved in normal cell cycles. These compounds have very specific sites of action.

Conclusion

We stand at the brink of an herbal revolution that will bring us new cures, improved diagnostic materials, and lower priced drugs with fewer side effects. In addition, the technology will enable manufacturers to standardize herbals in order to ensure optimum efficacy.

The miracle is not only that the herbs will help to cure and prevent diseases that have plagued mankind; doses of these herbs will be standardized with a high degree of accuracy. Perhaps most importantly, those who looked at the nutriceutical industry with skepticism will have all the answers they need.

Thanks to signal transduction technology, the health-giving properties of a variety of natural remedies will be elucidated. At the very least, the technology will provide rational support for the use of dietary supplements because it will demonstrate a molecular effect that can be beneficial to health. Previously, these supplements may have been promoted on more tenuous grounds.

The conflict between proponents of herbal medicine and the medical establishment is coming to an end. Herbal medicines are about to embark on a new era of respectability. The anecdotal evidence so long scoffed at by scientists will no longer be the sole documentation for efficacy.

The practice of modern medicine can now be enhanced by the best of ancient herbal remedies. The words of Paracelsus seem to be echoing through the ages. Almost five hundred years after he spoke, we finally have the opportunity to do as he asked: Let Nature be the physician. The miracle herbs are upon us.

5

The Lure of Botanicals

Deep in the valleys of India, high in the mountains of China, along the banks of the Amazon in South America, you will find no pharmaceutical sales representatives. Here, indigenous peoples still practice the medicine handed down to them by their ancestors. One is far more likely to deal in herbs than in chemicals. The plant world, however, does not exist separate from the chemical; the two are, in fact, inexorably interwoven.

Scientists today understand that plants are actually biosynthetic laboratories. The chemicals they create include compounds such as carbohydrates, protein, and fats. Many of the chemicals found in plants can exert a physiological influence; these chemicals include compounds such as glycosides, alkaloids, and volatile oils, which are known as phytochemicals. One of the first phytochemicals to be commonly used in Western medicine was a glycoside found in an herb called foxglove (*Digitalis purpurea*).

Finding Out About Phytochemicals

In the later part of the eighteenth century, an English physician combined his love of botany with his practice of medicine. Dr. William Withering was frequently called upon to treat dropsy, a condition now called edema. It is characterized by an abnormal accumulation of fluid and is usually caused by the heart's inability to pump blood at sufficient pressure, a condition known as congestive heart failure. Discovering that one of his patients had recovered from dropsy after taking a "secret potion," Dr. Withering set out to investigate the ingredients.

Out of the twenty herbs in the concoction, foxglove, or *Digitalis purpurea*, seemed a likely candidate. Dr. Withering soon found that the leaves of this plant afforded the most potent action. He dried them, ground them to powder, and administered a grain or two to patients. The swellings disappeared. After publishing his findings in 1785, Dr.

73

Withering became an international celebrity. Scientists today know that foxglove contains a cardiac glycoside that can increase the force of systolic pressure, heart contractions that drive blood through the aorta and pulmonary artery.

From a chemical point of view, glycosides are organic compounds that contain a nonsugar component and a sugar component. In most glycosides, glucose is the sugar. In plants, glycosides have regulatory, protective, and sanitary functions. Because of their regulatory role, glycosides are often therapeutically active. Herbal remedies containing glycosides include cathartics such as senna, rhubarb, and cascara sagrade. In wintergreen, the glycoside called gaultherin provides the analgesic methyl salicylate.

Medicinal phytochemicals are often alkaloids. These chemicals get their name from their alkaline qualities; with a pH greater than 7, they are caustic and basic in their chemical reactions, have a bitter taste, and always contain a nitrogen atom. Alkaloids appear to be secondary compounds — those that are not required for a plant's essential functions. More than four thousand alkaloids are known, ranging from caffeine to cocaine.

In the early 1800s, a pharmacist's assistant in Germany isolated the compound that gave opium its power; he called it *morphium,* known today as morphine. Once opium was understood to be an alkaloid, the search for plants containing these phytochemicals was on. Very soon, many pure alkaloids in plants were found — strychnine, used as a rodent poison and central nervous system stimulant, in 1817; caffeine in 1820; nicotine in 1828; atropine, traditionally used to dilate the pupils of the eyes and as an antispasmodic, in 1833; and cocaine in 1855.

Phytochemicals also include volatile or essential oils. These are the odorous principles found in any number of plant parts. They are called volatile because they evaporate readily when exposed to air. The name *essential* refers to the belief that they are the "essence" of the plant. In plants, volatile oils act as hormones, regulators, and catalysts. These oils are emitted from roots and aerial parts to fight off insects and inhibit the growth of competing plants. People have long availed themselves of plants' ability to ward off insects: Oil of citronella is a highly regarded insect repellant. In addition, essential oils derived from peppermint, dill, caraway, and fennel have long been known to be capable of relieving a variety of gastrointestinal symptoms. Essential oils may also aid in fat digestion by stimulating contractile activity in the gallbladder, thereby allowing the free flow of bile.

Volatile oils also play a role in the fertilization of plants. Unfertilized flowers can emit a strong fragrance for a week or until the flower dies. When impregnated, the flower loses its odor in less than thirty minutes. Aromatherapy derives its benefits from this property of volatile oils. We know that the sense of smell can evoke a host of memories and emotions. Most people do not, however, know that the olfactory nerves are directly connected to a primitive part of the brain sometimes called the reptilian brain, which regulates activities related to sex, hunger, and thirst. Proponents of aromatherapy believe that the scent puts a person in natural equilibrium, thus diminishing problems in various tissues. Aromatherapy is also a proven stress reducer.

Most essential oils are colorless and lighter than water. Unlike other oils, they do not leave greasy stains. Although they do not become rancid, essential oils do oxidize and resinify; they must be kept in dark, sealed containers. Volatile oils are usually obtained by water and/or steam distillation.

New Fields of Study Revolutionize Herbal Medicine

The roles of a few plant and animal chemicals have been recognized for more than three thousand years. Ancient warriors in the jungles of South America, for instance, used the poisons from plants and frog skins on their arrow tips, but only in the past four decades has the field of chemical ecology come to prominence. People involved in this field are now teaching us how various organisms use special chemicals in interacting with their environments. One of the most exciting developments is the use of natural chemicals as a safer approach to controlling pests.

We have already seen how essential oils act as insect repellants. In addition, St. John's wort contains a chemical called hypericin that is activated by sunlight. Insects that eat the plant during the day ingest the hypericin, which is then absorbed from the insect's gut. Molecules of the chemical reach the insect's outer surface, and when the insect is exposed to sunlight, the chemical poisons it.

According to a July 1996 article in *Chemical and Engineering News*, pest control is just one area in which chemical ecology has "sparked a revolution." Medical research and our understanding of animal communication have also been enhanced by the studies. Even world diplomacy is being affected.

The World Health Organization has set "Health for All by the Year 2000" as its priority goal. Achieving this goal will require the use of techniques from traditional medical systems in all countries. Scientists the world over are now researching these traditional medicines, which are frequently botanicals.

In 1993, the National Institutes of Health, the National Science Foundation, and the U.S. Agency for International Development launched the International Cooperative Biodiversity Groups (ICBG) program. Through the ICBG, investigators are searching Latin America and Africa for naturally occurring substances that can be used to treat or prevent diseases such as cancer, infectious diseases including AIDS, cardiovascular diseases, malaria and other parasitic diseases, and mental disorders. Many of those involved in the program believe that it should be expanded to consider end products other than drugs. The herbs being studied can also yield veterinary and agricultural products, cosmetics, flavors, and fragrances.

In Suriname, Africa, and especially Peru, researchers have invested heavily in the ethnobotanical approach; ethnobotany is the study of how different cultures use plants. Ethnobotanists decide which plants to collect and investigate by speaking with traditional healers and indigenous peoples.

The researchers also turn to ethnomedicine, which explains how a material is prepared and administered and describes the pertinent rituals or ceremonies, if any exist. If this seems foolish, consider the following case, in which ethnomedicine provided a solution to a problem scientists couldn't solve.

Scientists had been working with the active alkaloid in a plant used as an antimalarial. Although the alkaloid was active in vitro, it didn't work when injected into animals. The chief pharmacognosist associated with the project decided to speak with a traditional healer. The healer could not understand why the researchers injected the substance because she administered it by mouth. Thus, the researchers realized that the drug needs to be metabolized in an animal system. According to the pharmacognosist, if the researchers had been "too arrogant" to consider the ethnomedical facts, they might have abandoned a very worthwhile project.

In November 1994, an article entitled "Chemical Prospectors Scour the Seas for Promising Drugs" appeared in *Science*. The author notes that researchers today are "as intrigued by new natural pharmaceuticals as fifteenth-century explorers were by spices." Some natural pharmaceuticals have already proven to be beneficial.

In early April 1997, a lengthy cover article in *Chemical & Engineering News* was entitled "Seeking Drugs in Natural Products." In discussing comments made by a vice president of screening at Bristol-Myers Squibb, the article's author, A. Maureen Rouhi, says, "Even with rational drug design, chemical synthesis, and combinatorial chemistry, drug companies still need to go back to nature." Brian G. Schuster, a physician and pharmacologist from Walter Reed Army Institute of Research, is quoted as saying, "What the natural products offer us are whole new classes of compounds that haven't been available before." Consider that approximately ten thousand natural products from leaves, bark, and other plant matter are being tested annually at a single laboratory — the National Cancer Institute's lab in Frederick, Maryland.

At the University of Illinois, the College of Pharmacy is home to a collaborative research program funded by the National Cancer Institute. The program's director, John Pezzuto, says that six hundred plants have already been tested for medicinal properties and another four hundred are slated for testing before the program ends. He says that, so far, "The big surprise was resveratrol."

Found in more than seventy common plants such as grapes and peanuts, resveratrol was tested in tumor-bearing mice. The compound was effective in three stages of cancer: the initiation stage during which DNA is mutated; promotion, in which the affected cell becomes cancerous; and progression, when cancer cells form a tumor and spread.

Ancient Wisdom Offers New Hope

The American public's burgeoning interest in herbal medicines has led to increased interest in traditional Chinese medicine. Evidence of this can be seen in increasing foreign sales of traditional Chinese medicines, which are expected to double to more than $2 billion by the year 2000.

According to Wallace Sampson, M.D., clinical professor of medicine at Stanford University School of Medicine, traditional Chinese herbs yield remedies that are sometimes safe and effective, but on occasion are inert and at other times dangerous. He says, "It is difficult if not impossible, in most instances, to tell which concoctions belong in which of these categories." Researchers are now turning the impossible into an everyday reality; signal transduction technology permits them to discover exactly which "concoctions" are safe and effective.

Paul Kurtz, Ph.D, a professor emeritus of philosophy at the State University of New York at Buffalo says, "Openminded physicians everywhere would welcome any treatment that could benefit their patients, regardless of its origins, providing it can demonstrate its value in properly controlled clinical trials." One traditional Chinese medicine is about to go into clinical trials for the treatment of Alzheimer's.

The drug was discussed in a March 1997 issue of the *Journal of the American Medical Association,* which reported that an alkaloid compound called huperzine A had been found in the traditional Chinese herbal medicine *qian ceng ta.* Huperzine A is an inhibitor of acetylcholinesterase. This enzyme is found in nerve synapses and plays a role in the functioning of the central nervous system.

Long used to fight fever, this traditional herbal medicine is prepared from the moss *Huperzia serrata.* The purified drug has been used in China as a prescription medication for the treatment of dementia for several years. Approximately ten thousand people have been treated with the drug with no evidence of toxicity. If it proves effective against Alzheimer's, traditional Chinese herbs will have moved firmly into Western medicine. Even if it does not prove effective, other Chinese herbs are already proving beneficial.

By the early 1980s, researchers had isolated and purified andrographolide, the active bitter principle of the *Andrographis paniculata* leaf. The amount of andrographolides in the leaves and stems of the herb varies according to season and region. In a given region, the highest yield of andrographolide is attained before the plant blooms. The leaves of *Andrographis paniculata* were found to have the highest concentration of andrographolide, and the seeds the lowest. In addition, stigmasterol, a steroid, has been isolated in one fraction of this herb.

When *Andrographis paniculata* is subjected to the most sophisticated modern technology, the herb leaps into the arena of modern wonder drug. Indian pharmacologists using high pressure liquid chromatography have been able to standardize the herbal drug kalmegh, which consists of the dried leaves and tender shoots of the plant. In experiments using signal transduction technology, extracts of *Andrographis paniculata* have been shown to alter processes that interfere with the cell cycle. Interference with the cell cycle is at the root of the development of cancer or infection with viruses such as HIV-1. Researchers now believe that andrographolides can dramatically enhance immune system functions such as white blood cell production, release of interferon, and the activity of the lymph system. Andrographolides may also have some interesting properties in cancer therapy (see Chapter 7).

Reports from China, Thailand, and India have often described the use of *Andrographis paniculata* to help the body fight off invading organisms, such as bacteria. Many clinical trials have been reported, but they usually involved only small numbers of subjects, and some trials lacked controls. The sheer number of studies of the herb's effects on sick people and the consistency of the results still indicate that *Andrographis paniculata* has important therapeutic effects. Furthermore, practitioners of ethnomedicine frequently report that the herbal preparations have fewer side effects than synthetic drugs. Therefore, many establishment scientists have researched the medicinal value of the herbs, particularly since the 1970s, when *Andrographis paniculata*'s antibacterial effect and its effect on immunologic functions were first reported.

Scientists began their studies by investigating the safety of the herb. In traditional Chinese medicine, *Andrographis paniculata* has long been perceived as safe. Formal toxicological studies in animal models and in animal and human clinical trials confirmed that andrographolide has very low toxicity (see Appendix A). Rats and rabbits that received extracts of *Andrographis paniculata* once a day for seven days showed no adverse effects. Body weights were not affected; all blood, liver, and kidney tests were normal; and the animals remained energetic. When mice were given very high doses of the extracts, they became lethargic, but none of the animals died and there was no damage to major organs. At even higher doses, 50 percent of the animals died.

Some people who use the herb experience dizziness and heart palpitations, but reports of these side effects are extremely rare. Large oral doses are occasionally associated with stomach disturbances and poor appetite; vomiting sometimes occurs because of the extremely bitter taste. In addition, there have been some reports of hives and other allergic reactions following injection of raw *Andrographis paniculata* products. One possible drawback to use of the herb is a poorly defined antifertility effect that has been seen in some animal models but has not been repeated in humans. (It should be noted that many powerful synthetic drugs have potential antifertility effects.)

When high doses of *Andrographis paniculata* were administered to animals, production of both egg and sperm was interfered with. In addition, large doses brought about spontaneous abortions.

The effects of *Andrographis* on reproductive capacity in animals are not unique; such effects have been noted with many herbal extracts. Dietary supplements, in particular those made from herbs, are therefore best avoided in pregnancy. In research conducted around the world over the past twenty years, *Andrographis paniculata* has been shown to:

- relieve pain
- lower blood pressure
- reduce fevers
- control diarrhea
- reduce inflammation
- prevent blood clots
- prevent the development of ulcers
- halt the spread of viruses
- protect the liver
- lower blood sugar

In addition, test after test has confirmed that the herb has low toxicity in humans at doses recommended as dietary supplements.

One may well question how a single herb can have such a wide variety of beneficial effects. In fact, some people claim it is the mark of a charlatan to assert that a substance is a panacea. It appears, however, that the chemical constituents of *Andrographis paniculata* bring about successful clinical outcomes in a myriad of conditions, such as influenza, coronary artery disease, dysentery, gastric distress, and colds because of three simple properties: The herb's chemical constituents are antioxidative, immunostimulatory, and sedative. Many other herbs may have these miracle properties.

Medical Treasures of the Rain Forests

Andrographis paniculata is just one of the "miracle herbs" currently being researched. We now realize that scientists have examined less than 1 percent of the world's plants for medicinal activity. Because the greatest concentration of higher plants is in the tropics, researchers are turning — or perhaps returning — their attention to the rain forests of Central and South America.

Earth is a varied place — deserts, mountain slopes, riverbanks, savannahs. Each area is unique in its geography, climate, and natural inhabitants, with specialized areas referred to as "life zones." One such zone is a rain forest, a tropical forest with annual rainfall of at least one hundred inches.

Rain forests began to develop in Africa, Asia, and Central and South America about one hundred million years ago. For millions of years after that, rain forests encircled the globe. Within these dense evergreen forests, hundreds of thousands of species of life — perhaps half the species of the planet — live together, depending on each other for survival. Today, rain forests are roughly equal to the area of the continental United States; most of the original forests are archipelagos, or large groups of islands. Approximately 99 percent of a rain forest is plant life. At the foot of the Andes in Ecuador, perhaps as many as fifty thousand different species live.

From the time of Columbus to the mid-nineteenth century, men flocked to the Amazon jungle to investigate the plethora of exotic new life forms. Botanists, naturalists, and anthropologists were united by their curiosity. It did not take long for them to learn that their best source of information was the shaman.

In parts of South America, shamanisim is practiced today much as it was millennia ago. The South American shaman is initiated through inheritance or quest with his power coming from direct contact with the spirit world. He drinks a hallucinogenic brewed from a vine, and this transports him to heaven. The shaman cures people whom the spirits have made ill. He and his followers believe that cure involves "sectioning" magical objects out of an ill person's body. In some cases, the shaman can accomplish this goal by administering plant medicines to patients.

The shaman is not simply an herbalist. Under the influence of hallucinogenic plants, the shaman experiences visions that allow him to intervene in the spirit world. Whether the shaman administers plants directly or uses them to contact the spirit world, botanicals are an important part of his medical practice. Throughout history, botanicals have provided men with cures, but sometimes these cures eluded men for generations.

Finding Medicinals in the Rain Forest

When the Spanish conquered Peru in 1533, they were impressed with the Indians' sophisticated pharmacopoeia. Astounded by potent vegetable potions that the shaman swallowed to induce hallucinations, the Spanish marveled at samples of wound-healing saps and fever-reducing herbs. Within sixty years of the conquest, herbs, barks, and resins from Peru were being marketed in Spain. One of the most important medicines ever discovered came out of the rain forest in the seventeenth century.

Malaria had long plagued civilization; it is referred to in the Old Testament as *kadachas*, a term still used in Israel. Hippocrates wrote such a graphic description of one malaria epidemic that little more of importance was added for two millennia. In Vedic medicine, malaria was the most dreaded disease. Up to two thirds of the deaths in India at various times were caused by malaria. Predominant in autumn, it was called *takman* after the demon that was supposed to cause it. One hundred years ago, in Hyderabad, India, an Englishman finally discovered that the malaria parasite is transmitted by the *Anopheles* mosquito.

Throughout ancient and medieval history, the disease struck vast numbers, and there was no cure or effective treatment. The discovery of cinchona bark and its action on malaria changed all that.

In 1630, the Spanish conquerors of Peru found that the natives used the bark of a local tree to overcome fevers. The aborigines of Peru called the bark *quina quina* or "holy wood." One tale has it that the Quichua Indians had discovered the bark's effectiveness by watching jaguars. When struck by fever, the big cats cured themselves by gnawing on the bark of the quina tree.

In 1638, the countess of Chinchon, wife of the governor of Peru, was in

Lima, where she became ill with malaria. Her physician decided to try the bark treatment. He and the countess journeyed to the city of Loja, where her fever abated after she drank the brew. In 1640, the Viceroy del Chinchon brought the bark to Europe. As the story of the countess's recovery spread across Western Europe, the bark became known as cinchona. Some discount this tale as mere myth, although Carolus Linnaeus, eighteenth-century founder of the modern classification system for plants and animals, did give the name Cinchona to the fever tree in honor of the countess. Unfortunately, his spelling was not as good as his taxonomic classification system.

Powdered cinchona bark was used to treat malaria until two pharmacy professors in Paris isolated the active ingredient — quinine — in 1820. The demand for quinine was astounding. In 1850, nine tons of it were used in British India alone. The wide availability of the drug probably changed the course of world history; without it, European colonization of tropical countries might not have been possible.

The trend toward synthesizing the drug was firmly established during World War II, when Java's cinchona plantations were taken over by the Japanese. With its supplies of antimalaria drugs cut off, the Allies poured almost as much time and effort into the development of a new antimalarial as they did into the development of penicillin. In 1944, two American scientists finally synthesized chloroquinine.

Until the late 1960s, chloroquine was the preferred drug for treating malaria, since it is both inexpensive and readily available, however, strains of malaria resistant to chloroquine soon began to appear. Perhaps as many as thirty million cases of drug-resistant malaria were reported in India in 1977; in Ibadan, Africa, 45 percent of the malaria cases are resistant to chloroquine. Once again, the only effective treatment proved to be quinine. Renewed demand led to the planting of new plantations.

In the Rain Forests of Peru

Some of the earliest and most sophisticated herbal remedies were used by the Incas and other indigenous tribes of South America. Several herbal remedies originated among the Callawayas, medicine men to the Incas who lived in the mountains northeast of Titicaca, Peru. Today, descendents of the Callawayas are engaged in the practice of herbal medicine in several regions of the Andes. They use a medical system that goes beyond herbal cures to include charms, bits of metal, minerals, and animal parts. These items serve a multitude of purposes, such as curing fever or preventing crop failure. When herbs and charms fail, the patients are referred to soothsayers, who prognosticate or prepare individuals for the inevitable.

Today's Callawayas sell herbs and paraphernalia that are said to attract partners, alleviate fear and anxiety, and provide a better earthly environment. Callawayan herbalists practice herbal medicine in several major South American cities where they have a significant following. In areas of the Andes where Callawaya medicine men originated, very few physicians or other practitioners of medicine can gain acceptance. The Callawayan influence has even led to some rejection of religion in rural locations in the Andes, perhaps implying the success of their system of ancient holistic care. A return to primitive medical systems or beliefs is not advocated by these authors, but the reader is prompted to note that the Callawayan medical system has survived for thousands of years, presumably because it has been, at least in part, effective.

One of the biggest problems in researching the use of herbal or botanical cures from the rain forests of Central and South America is that very few written records of herbal medicines exist. Indians, such as the Cabecars of Costa Rica, have a rich history of herbal medicine, but many secrets of their practice have been passed on orally from generation to generation. Recent reports from several Central American countries have revealed a wealth of botanical medicines that have been overlooked by modern civilization.

In the rain forests of Costa Rica, for instance, more than two hundred putative plant extracts that act as medicinals have been identified. Dr. Rafael Angel Ocampo of the academic institution Centro Agronomico Tropical de Investigacion y Ensenanza (CATIE) has made major contributions to the identification and preservation of medicinal plants in Central America. Dr. Holt has reviewed Dr. Ocampo's works and spent time with him at CATIE.

Dr. Ocampo's studies of ethnobotany have revealed a crisis situation in the preservation of medicinal plants in Central and South America. Many plants identified as possible sources of extracts for the treatment of cancer, pulmonary disease, and recalcitrant infections are disappearing from the rain forest. Some plants with the greatest medicinal potential are regarded as weeds and are often destroyed by agricultural progress, crop planting, or landscaping.

In an attempt to combat this potential loss of medicinal plants, Professor Jorge Arce of CATIE has developed a special garden of medicinal plants where more than thirty species are grown organically to propagate and protect them. This garden contains many medicinal plants that have a history of use for curing a variety of diseases. During Dr. Holt's visit to this botanical asylum, he was able to sample several plants, including intriguing herbs that were natural sweeteners, antianxiety drugs, and decongestants. The sad reality is that the efforts of Jorge Arce and Rafael Ocampo are poorly supported by government or public funds. Some species of rain forest or tropical plants with healing or curative properties will undoubtedly be lost without greater support to rescue our ecological treasures.

The Quest for Curare

Along the Amazon, a people called the Yameos covered the points of their arrows with a poison that killed in less than a minute. They called it *ourari*. The first Europeans to encounter the poison were at a loss as to its source. Medicine men guarded the formula, cloaking its preparation in elaborate ritual. Some believed that the poison was compounded of thirty different herbs and roots. Then in 1799, Baron Von Humboldt located a source of this poison, now called curare, in Venezuela. He brought it back to Europe, where scientists found it worked by first stupefying and then asphyxiating its victims. Von Humboldt, however, failed to identify the vine used in the poison's preparation.

In the 1830s, a naturalist from England found the Macousis people in British Guiana making curare from the lianas vine. Naming the vine *Strychnos toxifera*, the naturalist became the first European to pinpoint the botanical source of curare. The poison was not fully understood until well into the twentieth century.

By 1930, it had been hypothesized that at the junctions between nerve and muscle, a row of nerve cells faces a row of muscle cells across a gap. An electronic impulse from the central nervous system incites nerve cells to release neurotransmitters that crisscross the gap, causing muscles to expand or contract. Scientists believed that curare blocked the receptors on the muscle cells so that neurotransmitters were not received and skeletal muscles shut down.

In 1935, a British chemist finally isolated the active ingredient, a crystalline alkaloid that he called *∂*-tubocurarine chloride. Scientists then sought quantities of the botanical to make pure extracts that might be used to treat convulsive diseases such as epilepsy, rabies, and multiple sclerosis. Supplies were, however, limited and of varying quality. Furthermore, suppliers — individuals who ventured deep into the rain forests — were not always reputable or reliable. Drug companies were loathe to deal with these people, just as they may be loathe to deal with some segments of the modern dietary supplement industry.

At this time, an American named Richard Gill was working as a rancher in the Ecuadorean Andes. Previously a medical student, Gill had always been intrigued by local medicines. When he was diagnosed with multiple sclerosis, a physician told him about a poison used by the Indians in the Amazon. It had a powerful relaxing effect on muscles, which neurologists thought had potential for treating multiple sclerosis. Unfortunately, the medical community could not get supplies for experimentation. Gill immediately recognized the poison as curare and set out on a search for an appropriate source.

In 1938, having secured financial backing from a Massachusetts businessman, Gill returned to Ecuador. He eventually convinced local medicine men to show him how the poison was prepared. Stems from three types of vines — *tonispa pala ango, lamas ango,* and *tonispa* — were bruised, boiled, and strained with elaborate ritual. Drawing upon the ancient tradition of the shaman as observer, Gill watched the preparation ceremony at several different locations. Finally he identified the potent vine as *tonispa pala ango,* the only vine used in every ritual he had watched. Gill returned to America in 1939, his baggage filled with the secret of curare and bundles of hope.

Although ensuing research on the therapeutic effects of curare yielded no evidence that it was effective against spastic diseases, it was not destined to fade into obscurity. In 1942, Harold Griffith, a Canadian physician and anesthesiologist, found that when curare was used in conjunction with a general anesthetic, muscular relaxation was more consistent and more complete. Patients given the combination required less anesthetic for chest and abdominal surgery, decreasing the dangers of such procedures.

Recognition of curare's benefits helped to usher in a new era for rain forest medicinals. Interest in South American botanicals was heightened by the discovery of a manuscript that had been hidden for 350 years. Written by a Spanish botanist in 1552, it contained a multitude of color illustrations and detailed the *materia medica* of the Aztecs. More than 250 plants are discussed in great detail; among them is the yam.

Dried yam root was soon being used in the United States to treat coughs and to induce perspiration and vomiting. Then, in Mexico City, the yam was shown to yield progesterone. This natural hormone could sell for just a few dollars a gram, while the previously used synthetic had cost $80 per gram. Drawing its name from *synthesis* and *Mexico,* a major pharmaceutical company (Syntex) was set up to manufacture and sell the natural progesterone. The company soon became a world leader in steroid chemistry and is still flourishing today.

Syntex was not the only company to profit from native botanicals. In 1952, E. R. Squibb and Sons (now Bristol Myers-Squibb) began marketing Raudixin. A treatment for hypertension, the drug contained an extract from the root of *Rauwolfia serpentina.* In India, the plant had long been used to treat nervous disorders, insanity, and snakebite. Reserpine, the active ingredient, was eventually isolated and is now used in numerous antihypertensive and psychiatric drugs.

Between 1950 and 1965, drug companies sent hundreds of researchers to South America and Africa in search of profitable medicinals. Unfortunately, botanicals vary biologically and chemically, which resulted in varied experimental results. Supplies were subject to natural disasters, poor transportation, and the vagaries of local politics. Synthetics began to look more and more appealing. That is, until the success of taxol, a successful treatment for ovarian cancer derived from the bark of the Pacific yew tree. Fears that there could not possibly be enough bark to provide treatment over the long haul led to the production of taxol from semisynthetic processes. Still, the die had been cast. Once again, drug manufacturers are actively looking to nature.

In the Rain Forest Today

Sometimes it seems that the search for rain forest medicinals has reached an almost fever pitch. Pharmaceutical companies are eagerly seeking out medicinals that have been used in the Amazon River basin since time immemorial. In 1954, Richard Evans Schultes returned to the United

States after spending thirteen years in South America. During most of that time, he had been searching out medicinal and hallucinogenic plants in the Amazon, a jungle that stretches from the Atlantic coast of Brazil to the Andes on the west coast of Peru and Chile. He brought with him twenty-four thousand plant specimens, two thousand of which are used by traditional healers. These specimens are still being studied at Harvard.

Investigators also hope to soon manufacture a topical prepared from the bark of a rain forest tree. In Peru, the natives remove the bark from the lowest part of a certain type of tree trunk. Where the bark had been, a type of resin appears. When spread on infected areas of the skin, the substance eliminates dermatological fungi such as ringworm.

Another bark from the rain forest is making headlines. Brazilian Indians have used the bark of the towering *Tabuia avellanedae* tree as a medicinal for hundreds of years. Native therapeutic uses include the treatment of colitis, dysentery, diarrhea, fever, and various cancers. Called *palo d'arco*, or "bow wood," by the natives, the herb is — somewhat mistakenly — known as *pau d'arco* in the United States and Europe. In these countries, the bark's medicinal properties have been studied for one hundred years or so. The bark has been proven to have antibacterial, antiviral, antiparasitic, anticancer, and anti-inflammatory properties.

In 1882, the first active constituent — lapacho — was studied. It was found to have a large range of quinones, a class of aromatic compounds. Used in tanning and photography, quinones are an essential part of vitamin E and coenzyme Q. Researchers were soon able to demonstrate that lapacho has antimicrobial activity. It was found that lapacho can increase oxygen supply at the local level, destroying bacteria, viruses, fungi, and parasites. Lapacho was shown to be effective against a large number of gram positive bacteria and fungi, such as *Staphylococcus*, *Candida albicans*, tuberculosis, and dysentery. It has also proven to be effective against the viruses herpes 1 and 2, and the influenza virus.

In 1968, studies conducted at the National Cancer Institute revealed that the active ingredient was very effective against tumors in rats. The study was abandoned due to fear of toxicity, though the head of the study later reported that the toxicity fears were groundless. In fact, the literature does not include significant reports of human toxicity despite the bark's abundant use over the past decade in Japan, Europe, South America, and the United States.

Americans today purchase the bark under the names *La pacho, taheebo, tecoma,* and *ipe roxo.* It has been found that the whole bark has more therapeutic value than extracts do. To get the full benefit of the whole bark, a decoction must be prepared. This is achieved by boiling 1 teaspoon of the bark in two 8-ounce cups of water for ten minutes. A daily dose consists of 1 cup of the decoction, two to eight times per day. In extract form, the recommended dose is 15 to 30 drops, two to eight times a day.

In addition to palo d'arco, other rain forest medicinals hold promise as cancer treatments. Researchers at the University of Illinois believe that a compound extracted from *Cassia quinquangulata,* a legume from Peru, may soon provide a way to treat cancer. According to the National Cancer Institutes (NCI), approximately 70 percent of the botanicals useful in cancer treatment come from the rain forest. No wonder American pharmaceutical firms have paid the government of Costa Rica millions of dollars for the right to search out new drugs in its forests.

Conclusion

The plant kingdom is full of mysteries that we are daily learning to unravel. Hand in hand, the plant world and signal transduction technology will bring about a revolution in medicine.

The efficacy of miracle herbs like *Andrographis paniculata* will be confirmed. Alternative and allopathic medicine will finally join together and acknowledge a pluralistic or integrated approach. In the face of signal transduction technology, advocates of alternative medicine are embracing the validity of scientific experimentation. The modern pharmaceutical industry has already embraced scientific validity in drug and dietary supplement development strategies. Advocates of conventional or allopathic medicine are already oriented for that acceptance.

Signal transduction technology will permit investigators to see — and to prove — how various herbs can be used in the treatment of a myriad of ills. The most exciting uses may be in the treatment of cancer, heart disease, and AIDS. These diseases kill millions each year, yet cures are elusive, fraught with debilitating and dangerous side effects, and often prohibitively expensive. Tomorrow we will eliminate these problems, because today we stand at the brink of an entirely new treatment option: the miracle of herbs and botanicals.

6

Herbs Fight on Many Fronts

Headache. Sniffles. Runny nose. Watery eyes. It must be cold and flu season — again. Year in and year out, we are laid low and made miserable by the common cold. It seems no matter what marvels modern science brings to medicine, no one defeats the tiny virus that invades the upper respiratory tract. By now, we all know that there is no cure for a viral disease; antibiotics can only kill bacteria. When we have a cold, we must seek symptomatic relief — after all, what's so bad about feeling good?

The ill effect of feeling good is that much of the relief we gain carries side effects that we'd just as soon do without. Antihistamines frequently cause dry mouth; their use can make people nervous and, in some cases, nauseous. Cough medicines often make people drowsy and can cause inflammation of the mucous tissue in the mouth. In treating colds and flu, ancient practices offer modern man many benefits.

Advice From Native Americans

Long before the white man arrived in North America, native Americans depended on *Echinacea angustifolia*, known to early white settlers as rudbeckia. Considered a powerful alterative and antiseptic, the herb was used by both Native American and settler to treat typhoid, malaria, diphtheria, and the common cold. Echinacea's therapeutic potential was first reported in scientific literature in 1887 by John King, M.D. Then, in 1895, Lloyd Brothers Pharmacists, Inc., of Cincinnati began producing echinacea products. These products rapidly became the bestselling American medicinal plant preparation.

Soon, the "new" Americans began to look down on everything about "Indian" culture. Plant-based medicines were no exception. Nevertheless, the twentieth century brought with it increased interest in all things natural as well as respect for Native Americans. Again, plant-based medicines were no exception.

90

Since the 1970s, investigators have studied echinacea's ability to enhance the body's resistance to infectious agents. Today, three species of echinacea — *angustifolia, pallida,* and *purpurea* — are considered medicinal because of their ability to stimulate the immune system. Stimulation of the immune system means that antibodies and antitoxins are efficiently attacking invading organisms, such as viruses and bacteria. In certain tests, scientists saw that extracts of *Echinacea purpurea,* the most common species of the herb, increased destruction of bacteria and other foreign bodies. The herb is, therefore, commonly used to treat colds, flu, and yeast infections.

Researchers have identified several chemical compounds in the herb. Among these are volatile oils, caffeic acid derivatives, and polysaccharides. Echinacoside, a caffeic acid glycoside, was once considered a significant active ingredient, but researchers no longer believe it is involved in stimulating the immune system. Researchers now believe that the immunostimulatory activity depends on the combined action of several constituents. Some scientists believe that the herb stimulates the body's production of interferon, which activates immune system cells that cause the disintegration of invading organisms. Echinacea may also activate enzymes that block a virus's ability to duplicate and spread.

In 1992, two studies in Germany demonstrated that people who took echinacea recovered more quickly from colds and flu. In addition, the symptoms of the diseases were less severe. In another study, fifty-four people who were considered highly susceptible to colds were given 4 ml of *Echinacea purpurea* juice twice a day, while fifty-four susceptible people received a placebo. Researchers found that those who had taken the herbal juice reduced their risk of catching a cold by 36 percent. Those who did catch colds experienced only mild symptoms.

Recent studies have attempted to determine the optimum timing and dosage for echinacea in the treatment of flu. In one double-blind placebo-controlled trial, extracts of *Echinacea purpurea* were administered to one hundred eighty volunteers, half of whom received relatively low doses of the herbal extract while half received high doses. Volunteers who received a 900 mg dose of echinacea had statistically significant improvement in symptoms such as stuffy nose, sneezing, sore throat, and headache as compared with the placebo control group. A group of volunteers that received only a 450 mg dose did not show any significant improvement as compared to the control group.

Approximately three hundred clinical monographs on echinacea now exist. Although some of these indicate a lack of positive results or a poor risk-benefit ratio, these results were probably influenced by the materials used. It is apparent that much of the research published before 1988 was actually conducted with *Echinacea pallida*. In pharmacological and clinical studies conducted with *Echinacea purpurea,* test substances were derived from the expressed juice of the flowering plant, though the roots of *Echinacea purpurea* were often adulterated with *Parethenium integrifolium* roots, which are inactive.

The adulteration of echinacea during scientific testing highlights the importance of standardization. Consumers who require predictable health benefits from a botanical or herbal must purchase standardized products. By using them, you can be certain that you will get the same amount of active ingredient in each dose. Unfortunately, many dietary supplement purveyors are not manufacturers; they are unaware that many of their products are based on bulk purchases of inferior herbals or botanicals. In fact, the dietary supplement industry is quite rightly and repeatedly criticized for its lack of knowledge or certainty about the components of the products being sold. With all botanicals or herbals, standardization of the active ingredient is essential. Products from nonstandardized herbal sources or institutes are best avoided because the consumer cannot be certain of their actions. When using echinacea, do not be misled by the belief that a numbing sensation on the tongue indicates quality. This is a common misconception.

In addition to standardization of the active component, the form in which herbals such as echinacea are administered is important. In the case of echinacea, several people involved with herbal remedies recommend that you avoid ethanol extracts because the alcohol may destroy some active components. (See Chapter 11 for directions on juicing herbs.) In Germany, where there are more than three hundred echinacea products on the market, investigators recommend doses of 6 to 9 ml of the pressed juice of the fresh flowering *Echinacea purpurea* plant. Most experts in America believe that one should use 900 mg a day of solid dry powdered standardized extract to fight an infection, and they recommend that the herb be taken in three daily doses of 300 mg.

There are no reports of toxicity associated with the use of echinacea. In a few cases, the herb may cause mild stomach upset and/or diarrhea.

Herbalists caution those with autoimmune diseases such as leukosis, multiple sclerosis, tuberculosis, diabetes mellitus, and AIDS to avoid echinacea. People with compromised immune systems can, however, avail themselves of an herbal remedy that has even proven effective in the treatment of AIDS. This herb from the pharmacopoeia of ancient China is showing great promise in treating upper respiratory infections, and it seems to have an excellent safety profile.

From the East

Andrographis paniculata is one of the most popular medicinal herbs in China and India. This herbal agent is such an exciting and multifaceted health option that it is a prime example of the miracle of herbs. The herb has, for instance, emerged as one of the most important herbal advances in dealing with the common cold.

Andrographis paniculata grows in evergreen, pine, and deciduous forests and along the sides of roads. It appears to grow best in the tropical and subtropical areas of China and Southeast Asia, where it grows in all types of soil. It is the only plant that grows on the so called "serpentine soil" formations, which contain a great deal of aluminum, copper, and zinc. Some believe that the herb's ability to thrive in this environment is responsible for its ability to cleanse the human body of damaging substances such as toxins and microorganisms.

An annual plant, *Andrographis paniculata* grows from $\frac{1}{2}$ to 1 meter in height. The stem is quite quadrangular with lancelike leaves that vary in size up to 7.5 centimeters long and 2.5 cm wide. The corolla is 1 cm long, hairy, and rose-colored. Yellow brown square seeds are numerous. Because propagation is easily achieved by seeding, the herb is widely cultivated in India, Sri Lanka, Indonesia, and many regions of China, and also has been introduced to the West Indies.

Andrographis paniculata is commonly called chuanxinlian in China, where it is also known as kudanchao and zhanshejian. In India, it is commonly called kalmegh, and in traditional Thai medicine it is known as fah talai joan. Practioners in these areas use the herb to treat respiratory infections, pharyngitis, laryngitis, tonsillitis, pneumonia, herpes, enteritis, peptic ulcer, skin infections, and snakebites. It is also used to reduce fevers.

Andrographis paniculata contains active constituents called andrographolides. Four andrographolides constitute up to 2 percent in dry weight of the herb's leaves. These bitter crystalline substances have been known to exert potent health-giving benefits for centuries, and they have long been used to treat infections and fever and stimulate immune function.

A host of reports in traditional Chinese medicine clearly demonstrate that *Andrographis paniculata* can stimulate immune function. The herb appears to play a role in augmenting such immune functions as white blood cell production, release of interferon, and the activity of the lymph system. So successful is the herb in stimulating body defenses that it is used extensively in Scandinavian countries to prevent and treat common colds. Several uncontrolled and controlled clinical observations show that extracts of the herb are effective in reducing symptoms of colds and flu and preventing infection without untoward effects except for occasional allergies.

A multitude of clinical trials have indicated that *Andrographis paniculata* is highly effective in the treatment of respiratory infections. In the 1970s, andrographolides as well as pills made from the powdered whole plant were tested in the treatment of these infections, and it was considered to be 88 percent effective. In addition, when an andrographolide was used to treat 129 cases of acute tonsillitis, 65 percent of the patients improved. In addition, the pain and fever associated with pharyngotonsillitis in adults was successfully treated in 152 adults during a randomized, double-blind study.

When investigators used an andrographolide to treat forty-nine pneumonia patients, thirty-five patients exhibited positive changes in their conditions and nine were considered to be completely recovered. A similar study conducted with 111 pneumonia patients and 20 with chronic bronchitis and lung infections demonstrated an overall effectiveness of 91 percent. In 72 percent of the patients, fever subsided within three days; 40 percent had smaller areas of infection within one week; 79 percent had improved status within two weeks. A clinical trial involving 455 cases of infantile pneumonia showed an *Andrographis paniculata* product to be 90 percent effective, with an average of 3.1 days for body temperature to return to normal.

In Western Europe and in Scandinavia, *Andrographis paniculata* is widely used in a dietary supplement formulation to treat and prevent common colds. In 1992, clinical studies of an herbal formula containing extracts of *Andrographis paniculata* and *Acanthopanax senticosus* were begun in Sweden. The controlled, double-blind study conducted at the Occupational Health Center in Ulricehamn, Sweden, involved fifty patients. Researchers evaluated symptoms and clinical signs on the third or fourth day of the trial. Those using the preparation showed less fatigue, shivering, sore throat, muscular ache, rhinitis, sinus pain, and headache than those using the placebo. Test subjects had fewer sick days (.21) than patients who used the placebo (.96). Of those who used the preparation, 68 percent said they were completely recovered; only 36 percent of those who used the placebo believed themselves to have recovered.

In addition, 55 percent of those who used the preparation felt the course of the cold was "easier" than usual, as opposed to 19 percent who used the placebo. Researchers concluded that a daily dose of 1,200 milligrams of standardized extract can shorten the duration of an upper respiratory infection. These clinical observations of the beneficial effect of *Andrographis paniculata* coincide with work conducted by Paracelsian, Inc. At that company, researchers documented the immune-stimulating properties of andrographis through signal transduction experiments.

Turn to Green Fields

Echinacea and *Andrographis paniculata* are not the only botanicals that have been found effective in treating infections. Thyme has, for instance, been shown effective in the treatment of sinusitis, chronic respiratory infections, colds, flu, and sore throat. The volatile oil derived from the dried leaves and flower tops of *Thymus vulgaris* — thyme — is often used as an antiseptic, antifungal, and antibacterial. It is best to avoid thyme if you have high blood pressure.

Do remember that, as common as a cold may be, its complications can be serious. If you have a fever of more than 102° F. for three days or more, you should consult a health care practioner. Be sure to consult a physician if you have yellow or white spots in your throat or if the lymph nodes under your jaw or in your neck are swollen.

Fighting Fevers and Bacteria

Diseases far more serious than colds can also be treated with herbal medicines. Studies conducted in China and India demonstrated that fevers caused by such agents as endotoxin, *Pneumonococcus, Streptococcus,* typhoid, and paratyphoid are lowered by *Andrographis paniculata.*

In controlled laboratory tests, andrographolides were administered to rats with fevers. The extracts reduced the animals' fevers as effectively as aspirin.

Researchers now understand how andrographolides lower fevers. These extracts reduce muscle tone and dilate peripheral blood vessels, resulting in a lowering of fevers.

In tests conducted in Indonesia and reported in *Planta Medica,* andrographolides derived from *Andrographis paniculata* were shown to enhance white cells' ability to attack invading organisms like bacteria, viruses, and toxins. Several laboratories in China and India have also demonstrated that at low doses, *Andrographis paniculata* and the andrographolides enhance immune function, but at high doses lymph cells' ability to function is attenuated. The adverse effects of andrographis are often dose related, appearing only at high doses.

Researchers at the Central Drug Research Institute in Lucknow, India, continuously seek to develop chemotherapeutic agents from Indian medicinal plants. In several studies, they found that *Andrographis paniculata* extracts stimulate activity in the immune system. For example, tests in mice revealed that andrographolides increased the serum levels of an enzyme that destroys the cell walls of certain bacteria. Reporting in the *Journal of Natural Products,* the scientists concluded that *Andrographis paniculata* "is a potent stimulator of the immune response" and is capable of "enhancing both antigen specific and nonspecific responses."

Protecting the Liver

In Ayurvedic medicine, twenty-six different polyherbal formulations of *Andrographis paniculata* are used to treat liver disorders. Scientists recently demonstrated that extracts of *Andrographis paniculata* can protect the liver against a variety of damaging substances. In the 1980s it was shown that the leaf extract affords some protection against liver damage associated with alcohol consumption. Andrographolides have also showed a dose-dependent ability to protect the liver from damage caused by nonaspirin pain relievers (paracetamol and acetaminophen).

In Calcutta, researchers found that an extract from the leaves of andrographis can provide protection against liver damage caused by carbon tetrachloride or alcohol. (See Appendix A.) Carbon tetrachloride, a common degreaser for metals and a ubiquitous cleaning solvent in some countries, is a significant occupational hazard.

Andrographis paniculata products were administered to animals before they were exposed to various agents that could damage the liver. Lower levels of certain liver-associated enzymes and reduced damage to liver cells indicated that the products helped to protect the liver against toxic substances, including carbon tetrachloride and acetaminophen. Both of these extracts were found to be more effective as hepatoprotective agents than silymaron (milk thistle), which has long been used clinically.

One reason for this protective function may be that the glucoside components of certain *Andrographis paniculata* extracts act as strong antioxidants. Antioxidants prevent the formation of free radicals — particles that result from both natural processes and toxic substances in the body.

With certain toxic chemicals such as carbon tetrachloride and ethanol, or grain alcohol (the alcohol in whiskey), oxidation of cell membranes may play a prime role in the death of liver tissue. When the membrane oxidizes, the living envelope responsible for the cell's interaction with its environment can no longer transmit messages effectively. The membrane cannot absorb nutrients or process information, therefore it cannot combat underlying disease processes.

Preventing the oxidation of living cells — mopping up free radicals that cause cell damage — is currently a major issue in medicine. Certainly, the media has deluged us with information about antioxidants such as beta-carotene and vitamins C and E. When permitted to develop and grow, free radicals damage cells' DNA, leading to various diseases, including cancer.

Recent studies have, however, cast doubt on the concept that taking large doses of some antioxidants can protect against these diseases. In fact, in two trials involving beta-carotene taken by people at increased risk of cancer, the cancer and/or death rate actually increased. In a third trial involving twenty-two thousand healthy physicians who took beta-carotene regularly, no beneficial or negative effects were seen. Under these circumstances the promise of *Andrographis paniculata* may be even more appealing.

Andrographis paniculata can also protect the liver against infective hepatitis. A serious health risk the world over, hepatitis has no known cure and can eventually lead to liver cancer.

In one study, acute hepatitis was chemically induced in rats that were then given *Andrographis paniculata* extracts. (See Appendix A.) When blood samples and liver cells were subsequently examined, researchers found that biochemical signs of hepatitis had returned to normal. Studies with human subjects had similar results.

At the Institute of Medical Sciences at Banaras Hindu University in India, twenty patients displaying the jaundice of infective hepatitis received a decoction of *Andrographis paniculata* for twenty-four days at the rate of 60 ml per day. In all the patients, the color of urine and the inner surface of the eyelids returned to normal. Ninety percent of the patients regained appetite and 83 percent exhibited relief from depression. Ten subjects showed normal results on tests of liver function and experienced complete symptomatic relief; they were deemed cured. Four patients were relieved because liver function tests were normalized and they experienced considerable clinical improvement. In a similar test conducted in China with 112 cases of hepatitis, *Andrographis paniculata* was considered 83 percent effective. In other words, roughly eight out of every ten patients recovered.

Herbal Relief for Gastrointestinal Disorders

For centuries, essential oils from peppermint, dill, caraway, and fennel have been effectively used to relieve a variety of gastrointestinal symptoms. In 1986, the book *The Scientific Validation of Herbal Medicine* indicated that peppermint and fennel contain volatile oils and other constituents that absorb intestinal gas, calm an upset stomach, inhibit diarrhea or constipation, aid digestion, and prevent or remedy childhood colic.

Peppermint

Peppermint is one of the most underestimated herbals in medical practice. Peppermint is regarded as safe, but the Food and Drug Administration has quite surprisingly concluded that peppermint oil is ineffective for promoting the relief of digestive upset. This conclusion is amazing given the availability and endorsement of delayed release formats of peppermint oil as prescription and over-the-counter medicines for the treatment of irritable bowel syndrome in several European countries.

The essential oil of peppermint has been shown to have profound effects on gastrointestinal smooth muscle. Peppermint oil is a natural, calcium channel antagonist that causes relaxation of smooth muscle upon contact. Several well-conducted, double-blind, controlled clinical trials of peppermint in delayed release formulations show that peppermint is better than a placebo at relieving symptoms of irritable bowel syndrome.

Clinical studies in England have shown that peppermint oil in a delayed release capsule improves the acceptability of a colostomy. There are several hundred thousand colostomy patients in Western society and their biggest problem is diminished quality of life, often as a result of unwanted odor from the fecal contents of their colostomy bag. Some evidence exists that delayed release formulations of peppermint oil may regulate the function of the colostomy and effectively deodorize the contents of the colostomy bag.

The soothing effect of peppermint oil has been linked to the relief of flatulence and bloating. Gastric bloating may be associated with disturbance of upper gastrointestinal motor function, such as delayed gastric emptying. Relief is sometimes experienced after the belching of gas or the passage of flatus. It has been proposed that the passage of gas from the upper or lower digestive tract is facilitated by the breakup of intestinal foam.

Peppermint oil's mechanism of action appears to be related to a local stimulatory effect of essential oils on the gastrointestinal tract. This effect is frequently followed by a mild degree of local anesthesia. In addition, peppermint oil contains menthol, a chemical that resembles steroids. Rapidly absorbed from the upper portions of the small intestine when taken orally, menthol may modulate the gastrointestinal smooth muscle function.

Peppermint oil has been shown to have the ability to normalize gastrointestinal motor activity and relieve both spasm and flaccidity in the intestines. Furthermore, the oil has been found to inhibit or inactivate more than thirty microorganisms that have been implicated in digestive problems. Clinical reports propose peppermint oil as potentially useful in diarrhea caused by opportunistic infections of the bowel in AIDS patients and it may be useful in preventing travelers diarrhea.

Ginger

Today, many people find that peppermint tea has similar effects. In addition, ginger has become almost universally accepted as an antinausea treatment. The underground stem of the plant (rhizome) has been used in China and India for more than two thousand years to aid digestion and relieve nausea. In Germany and Denmark, ginger is currently approved for use in the treatment of motion sickness.

In 1982, an article in the British medical journal *Lancet* reported that people rotated in a tilted chair were less likely to feel sick if they took ginger. The herb's effect was reported to be greater than that of either Dramamine or a placebo. Later studies involving Danish naval cadets reinforced these results. Tests conducted at a hospital in England revealed that ginger was better at preventing postoperative nausea than the tranquilizer metoclopramide. Ginger has also been shown effective in curbing the nausea associated with chemotherapy and morning sickness.

It is recommended that people wishing to avoid motion sickness take two 500 mg capsules about half an hour before embarking. Because ginger seems to work almost entirely on the digestive system rather than on the brain, it can be used without incurring drowsiness or other side effects. There have been no reports of toxicity associated with ginger, which is a commonly used spice. It can, however, thin your blood; if you have bleeding problems or are taking anticoagulants, use ginger sparingly, if at all.

Andrographolides

In the traditional medical system of India, an *Andrographis paniculata* extract called alui has long been used to alleviate the discomfort of indigestion. Researchers were interested in learning whether andrographolides, extracts of *Andrographis paniculata,* would be effective in these cases.

To assess the effect of an androgapholide, it was administered to rats for three days; two hours after each dose, aspirin — which irritates the stomach lining, causing increased gastric secretions — was also administered. When the rats were autopsied, researchers found significant decreases in gastric juice secretion and total acid content relative to a control group. (See Appendix A.)

Eighty-five people suffering from chronic colitis were treated with a combination of *Andrographis paniculata* and the rhizome of *Rehmannia glutinosa*. Before retiring on fourteen consecutive nights, the participants used the liquid part of the mixture as an enema at doses of 100 to 150 ml. Of the subjects, sixty-one (72 percent) were considered clinically cured and twenty-two (26 percent) experienced symptomatic relief. Only two people did not respond to the treatment.

More Miraculous Effects

Andrographis paniculata has also been shown to prolong survival and postpone the respiratory failure caused by cobra venom. In several studies, *Andrographis paniculata* products were seen to produce a sedative effect. When administered to mice, these products were related to an increase in the duration of barbital-induced anesthesia. When used in conjunction with an *Andrographis paniculata* product, the anesthetic state was achieved even when doses of barbital drugs were reduced.

All andrographolides are also potent stimulators of gallbladder function. In animal experiments, rats and guinea pigs that received andrographolides for seven consecutive days evidenced an increase in bile flow, bile salt, and bile acids. Use of *Andrographis paniculata* might, therefore, decrease the probability of gallstone formation and might also aid fat digestion. Furthermore, andrographolides prevented the decreases in volume and content of bile that are often caused by acetaminophen toxicity.

In one study, *Andrographis paniculata* was compared with the clinical drug nitrofurantoin in the treatment of kidney inflammation caused by bacterial infection. The herb was found to be as effective as the standard drug but had fewer side effects.

Animal experiments have shown that extracts of *Andrographis paniculata* have antidiarrheal effects. Extracts were shown to be effective against *E. coli* endotoxin in rabbits and guinea pigs. An endotoxin is a component of the bacteria itself, often the cell wall. Used against the toxins that are the most common cause of neonatal diarrhea, an andrographolide was found to be superior to the commonly used antidiarrheal drug loperamide (Imodium). In high doses, this opium derivative can effectively stop bowel action. An alcohol extract of

Andrographis paniculata showed significant effects against the diarrhea associated with *E. coli* infections in a dose-dependent manner. In certain enterotoxin-induced cases of diarrhea, an andrographolide was superior to loperamide at 1 mg doses.

When ninety-four cases of acute bacterial diarrhea were treated with 500 mg of andrographolide in three dosing periods for six days, eighty patients were deemed cured. Seven other patients responded favorably to the treatment, and only seven patients had no response. Results were confirmed by stool samples. In another trial, *Andrographis paniculata* was used to treat 1,611 cases of bacterial dysentery; the success rate was reported to be 91.3 percent. Clinical tests of some fractions have not shown the herb to be effective in treating bacterial infections within the intestine, such as those caused by *Shigella dysenteriae,* a bacteria responsible for one severe form of dysentery.

It had been assumed that *Andrographis paniculata* products were effective against bacterial dysentery and diarrhea because they were antibacterial, but studies could not confirm reproducible antibacterial properties of either the herb or its products. No antimicrobial activity was seen in in vitro tests or in the serum of human volunteers given four different doses of the herb. The mechanism of the antidiarrheal and anti-infective properties of andrographis is not completely understood at this time.

The importance of an herbal treatment for diarrhea cannot be overemphasized. Diarrhea-type diseases are one of the top ten causes of death worldwide and are a leading cause of childhood mortality in developing countries. At present, there is no substance that can prevent the disease without side effects, and excessive use of antibiotics has resulted in antibiotic resistance. In developing countries, where the problem is practically catastrophic, an herbal remedy would be inexpensive and accessible enough to constitute a revolution in health care.

Health care would also be revolutionized by an herbal treatment for inflammatory conditions such as arthritis and allergies. Just consider that more Americans say they suffer from arthritis than from any other health problem. Arthritis and allergies cause great suffering and economic loss the world over. A cytokine called tumor necrosis factor, or TNF, is the force behind the biochemical cascade that causes inflammation. It normally protects the body against tumor development and infection, but when it is working abnormally, rheumatoid arthritis develops. Scientists at the University of Alabama in Birmingham have successfully treated rheumatoid arthritis with a drug that inhibits TNF, thereby controlling the cycle of inflammation.

In animal models, inflammatory markers were significantly reduced or relieved when andrographolides were administered. Researchers discovered that the anti-inflammatory effect of the various andrographolides differed. In all cases, however, the effect was found to be mediated by the adrenal glands: After removal of those, the anti-inflammatory effect disappeared. Additional studies confirmed that the anti-inflammatory action is due to *Andrographis paniculata*'s role in increasing synthesis and releasing the hormone that affects growth and the activity of the adrenal cortex.

Andrographolides were also tested in a clinical trial of tubercular meningitis patients. Normally such patients receive the synthetic drug rifampin. At the clinic where the *Andrographis paniculata* extract was tested, treatment with that drug normally entails a 22.5 percent fatality rate. When the patients received 50 to 80 mg/kg of solution of an andrographolide in addition to 20 mg of rifampin/kg for two months, the fatality rate dropped to 8.6 percent.

Conclusion

In an era when increasing numbers of disease-causing bacteria are showing resistance to drugs, the potential of andrographolides is vitally important. It has been reported that a number of common bacterial infections are often resistant to antibiotics. Researchers at Stanford University have now shown that some cases of chronic ear infections are caused by antibiotic-resistant bacteria. The authors of this book are not recommending substituting herbal remedies for antibiotics, but, at the very least, andrographis and other herbs could have a complementary effect on infections when used in conjunction with antibiotics. The possibility of combining effective natural remedies with effective synthetic medications opens up a new vista in medical treatment. This option is especially exciting, as it may help fight some drug-resistant diseases. In fact, the twenty-first century seems to promise a plethora of exciting options.

7

Herbal Miracles
in Cancer Therapy

The statistics are frightening:

- In 1990, six million people in the world died of cancer.
- Each year, more than one million Americans are diagnosed with some form of cancer.
- Cancer is the most common cause of death for children between the ages of five and fourteen.
- The incidence of most cancers is increasing.
- In the past thirty years, there has been a ninefold increase in the number of women who die annually from lung cancer.
- "Decades of research on new treatments have had little impact on reducing deaths due to cancer..." (*Chemical and Engineering News*, July 1997)

Despite amazing advances in technology, we seem to have made little progress in cancer treatment. Victims of the disease must still rely on treatments that involve cutting, burning, or poisoning their bodies: Surgery, radiation, and chemotherapy are their only options. No wonder so many seek answers in alternative medicine. Many alternative treatments, however, have not been subjected to rigorous scientific investigation. Hopefully, signal transduction technology will change these circumstances.

The genesis of cancer is a story of signals gone awry. Malignancies develop when cells do not respond to signals that normally limit growth. In addition, the cells that proliferate in malignant growths are undifferentiated; benign growths have functional, specialized cells.

Understanding the Cell Cycle's Role in Cancer

In the human body, many cells reproduce on a regular basis. Cells such as those in the testes, small intestine, and spleen divide frequently. Other cells — such as those in the brain, heart, and liver — have a low turnover. Runaway or uncontrolled cell replication anywhere in the body is the cornerstone of cancer. To understand how cellular proliferation can get out of control, one must first understand the cell cycle, which has been outlined in an earlier chapter. (See page 64.)

In recent years, scientists have made great strides in understanding this cycle and the causes of the cell cycle's running wild. They know, for instance, that the process of cancer often begins when a tumor suppressor gene is damaged. These genes normally act as "brakes," keeping new cell production at a moderate rate. In other cases, cancers begin when a mutator gene is damaged. Mutator genes normally protect the genes that are involved in cell division, but sometimes an oncogene is damaged. An oncogene gives cells the signal to divide, so damage to it can lead to an increased rate of cell division.

A number of different gene mutations are indications (markers) of human cancer. No matter which marker is present, changes in both chromosome number and structure occur. Other cancer markers can be seen in the cell cytoplasm, the semifluid substance outside the nucleus of a cell. When cells develop normally, each stage of development is accompanied by different cytoplasmic structures (organelles) with specialized duties related to the cell's functioning. When cancer blocks normal development, the organelles do not mature as they do under normal influences.

When scientists began to investigate the alterations in cytoplasmic development and in genes in malignant cells, they needed to know which changes were the cause and which were the effect. They noted that healthy, aging cells exhibit chromosomal alterations similar to those in malignant cells. It, therefore, appeared that changes in chromosomes may be secondary to the development of cancer.

Scientists now believe that chromosome stability depends on cytoplasmic differentiation, and control over both depends on the signals that the cell receives. As author and consultant Gerald B. Dermer, Ph.D., puts it, "Cancer is the result of a breakdown in the signaling mechanisms that control the orderly activity of genes in developing cells." Today, that signaling process has been elucidated.

Looking at the Signaling Process

The cell cycle is a series of events that culminates in division of a cell; the process begins again in two cells that can now be called the daughter cells. This is the normal process of cell reproduction.

Various mechanisms control the rate of cell reproduction. Without control, cells would reproduce too rapidly. It would be like putting your foot on the gas pedal of a car that had no brakes. Uncontrolled cell reproduction would cause a big mass or lump of cells to grow. Unfortunately, uncontrolled or unregulated growth does occur, and masses that we call tumors then develop.

If normal cell division is to occur, the various events in the process must receive the correct signal at the proper time. Scientists now know that the cell cycle is controlled by signals that move the events forward as well as other signals that act as brakes, halting cell replication when necessary.

Cell cycle signals can, in other words, be described as positive or negative regulators: CDKs are positive regulators that bring about cellular proliferation. On the other hand, there are proteins called tumor suppressor proteins and CDK inhibitory proteins that are negative regulators. These substances prevent progression of the cell cycle so that duplication of cells does not occur.

A large percentage of cancer cases have been associated with mutations of a tumor suppressor gene known as p53. In fact, among the 6.5 million people diagnosed with cancer annually, roughly 50 percent have p53 mutations in their tumors. As we have seen, if the p53 gene is mutated, unregulated cell growth can occur. (See Appendix A for additional information.)

Benefiting From Knowledge of the Cell Cycle

Using signal transduction technology, scientists found that p53 is activated by another gene, the p34, to halt cell replication. Abnormal p34 levels have been found in approximately 90 percent of breast tumor cells. Because scientists using signal transduction technology can find the p34 gene, its presence is now being used to diagnosis cancer.

In the hopes of producing antitumor agents, investigators are studying the signals that induce cell differentiation and proliferation. In April 1997, the University Medical Center at Stony Brook (Long Island, New York) announced its researchers had found an enzyme that may hold the key to breast cancer. According to molecular pharmacologist Craig Malbon, "a molecule known to be the gatekeeper for cell division is highly expressed in primary breast cancer. It is the signaling molecule responsible for switching a cell into proliferation." The molecule is MAP — mitogen-activated kinase — an enzyme that kicks off cell division. MAP is five to twenty times more abundant in breast cancer cells than in normal cells.

Molecular biologist Gary Johnson of the National Jewish Medical and Research Center in Denver says that the molecule MAP is part of a pathway that controls growth and is regulated by a gene called Ras, which is often damaged in cancer cells. A protein, Ras is understood to be one of the intermediate signals that enables cells to respond to external growth factors. To transmit its signal, Ras associates with a cell's plasma membrane. If Ras is mutated, the cell responds with uncontrolled growth. Ras breaks down in 30 percent of cancer cases, and mutated forms of the protein have been found in 95 percent of pancreatic cancers.

According to molecular biologist Gary Johnson, Malbon's work "identifies a viable target for new therapeutic approaches." Johnson points out, in fact, that there are drugs in the "very early phases of development that can inhibit this pathway. So if this finding can be shown to be related to many cancer cases, [the new drugs] could be very rapidly developed." At the University of Pittsburgh, for instance, researchers are developing drugs that will act directly on the Ras protein. Molecules designed by researchers at the university cross cell membranes and disrupt the processing of cancer-causing Ras.

Another compound that may be able to halt the spread of cancer comes from the herb *Andrographis paniculata*. Discovery of the herb's versatility is one result of unraveling the miracle of herbs.

Joining Modern Technology and Ancient Herbs

Now that researchers understand the path a cell travels to runaway growth, they are learning how to halt that growth by interfering with the signals that set it in motion. For instance, researchers know that CDK-1 mediates proliferation of the cells from which capillaries sprout. If CDK-1 does not send its signal, capillaries will not grow into the tumor mass. Without capillaries, the tumor's food supply will be restricted, waste products will not be removed, and the tumor will die. Armed with this knowledge, investigators began looking for practical applications. When modern technology joined with traditional Chinese medicine, the marriage produced amazing offspring.

When signal transduction technology was applied to studies of *Andrographis paniculata,* it became apparent that the herb had phenomenal anticancer powers. Japanese researchers — whose traditional medicine lends itself to the use of natural products — have led the research. One group of Japanese scientists reported dramatic evidence of the herb's ability to halt cell proliferation. These researchers cultured human stomach cancer cells in a medium that contained an *Andrographis paniculata* extract. After three days, there were 7.8 cells in the medium as compared to 120 cells in the control group. The extract certainly appears to have stopped cell replication.

In 1994, another group of scientists in Japan reported that an extract of *Andrographis paniculata* had shown potent differentiation-inducing activity on dividing cells. As you may recall, cells that proliferate in malignant growths are undifferentiated.

In a joint study conducted by the departments of chemistry at the University of Singapore and Tokyo Kyoiku University, tests were conducted on sarcoma cells. These cancers affect muscle, connective tissue, and bones and are usually very malignant. Three days after the researchers transplanted the sarcoma cells into the abdominal cavities of rats, intraperitoneal injections derived from crude plant extracts were administered. When the tumor samples were examined microscopically, *Andrographis paniculata* was found to inhibit the growth of tumors.

Laboratory tests in Buffalo, New York, revealed that an extract of *Andrographis paniculata* inhibits the growth of human breast cancer cells at levels similar to the commonly used drug tamoxifen. Proliferation of human breast cancer cells was inhibited over several days through the use of herbal extract concentrations almost equivalent to the concentration of various drugs commonly used to treat cancer.

In laboratory experiments, investigators have shown that andrographolide, a chemical component of *Andrographis paniculata,* can diminish CDK-1's ability to promote cell division. In other words, extracts of the herb can actually inhibit angiogenesis, the proliferation of blood vessels, thus bringing about the death of a tumor. Researchers around the world are actively investigating substances that can destroy or block the blood vessels that feed tumors. They believe that this strategy is superior to targeting tumor cells directly.

For many years, drug research has focused on destroying cancerous cells. This type of drug therapy can also harm or kill healthy cells, which is why chemotherapy has so many unpleasant side effects. Many researchers are now trying to destroy cells in blood vessels rather than in tumors. Because cells that line blood vessels are in direct contact with the blood, chemical agents can reach them more easily than cells of solid tumors. It should, therefore, be possible to use less powerful poisons. In addition, blood vessel cells are not likely to mutate and become resistant to therapy.

Some researchers are trying to interrupt the blood supply to tumors by blocking or occluding the blood vessels. They are trying to selectively initiate the series of events involved in blood coagulation. In experiments with mice, blood clot formation in the tumor vessels resulted in complete tumor regression in 38 percent of the animals. The events leading to coagulation are set in motion when certain enzymes initiate the conversion of inactive substances to their active state.

In addition to altering signals responsible for blood vessel growth, andrographolides, the active elements in the herb *Andrographis paniculata,* can be toxic to certain cells. Researchers in both Thailand and Japan have reported that leukemia cells are particularly sensitive to the cytotoxic effects of andrographolide. This research was confirmed by a project conducted jointly by the National Cancer Institute in Bangkok, Thailand; Khon Kaen University in Thailand; and the University of Sydney, Australia. Researchers found that andrographolide can destroy cells responsible for one type of lymphocytic leukemia and a certain type of skin cancer. At the end of the study, the researchers concluded that andrographolide's effectiveness in these diseases exceeds the values recommended by the protocol of the National Cancer Institute of the United States. A study of another traditional herb was recently conducted in China with similar results.

The Advantages of Herbal Cancer Treatments

During the Cultural Revolution in China, a team of physicians from Harbin Medical University was sent into the countryside. Their mission was to amass evidence that traditional Chinese medicine was superior to Western practices. The group found that locals had been using a broth to cure arthritis, skin disorders, and other conditions. Investigators soon purified the "secret ingredient": arsenic trioxide. They found that this arsenic compound brought about remission in more than 70 percent of the cases of acute promyelocytic leukemia. Five years later, almost half of these leukemia patients in one trial were disease-free. Although arsenic trioxide is toxic, the researchers were able to ameliorate the toxic effects by administering low doses intravenously.

Extracts of *Andrographis paniculata* are far less toxic than arsenic trioxide or most standard chemotherapeutic agents. Because of their toxicity, most chemotherapeutic agents have unpleasant and sometimes dangerous side effects. The much-touted breast cancer drug tamoxifen can, on rare occasions, be toxic to the liver. More often, use of the drug can cause retinal injury, pulmonary embolism, a drop in platelet count, nausea, and anorexia. A drug manual for nurses suggests they caution patients that "acute exacerbation of bone pain during tamoxifen therapy usually indicates the drug will produce good response."

Another cancer drug called cisplatin can cause anemia, seizures, and renal failure. The cancer drug etoposide can cause temporary hair loss, nausea, low blood pressure, and blood abnormalities. The botanical agent taxol is relatively safe in comparison to many synthetic drugs used in cancer chemotherapy.

Meanwhile, decades — if not centuries — of data collected in China indicate that *Andrographis paniculata* is well tolerated as an oral medication even when used for extended periods of time. When clinical trials using the herbal were conducted in China, oral doses of the extract were well tolerated, and dose regimens of three months or longer appeared reasonable. (See Appendix A for additional information.)

Observing Andrographis at Work

The studies we have just discussed gave early evidence supporting *Andrographis paniculata*'s role as a cancer therapy. This evidence was exciting, to say the least. Here was an all-natural, nontoxic, easily accessible material that might treat one of the most feared diseases known. One of the first human studies of the herb was reported in the *Journal of Chinese Medicine* in 1977. The study involved sixty skin cancer patients, including forty-one with confirmed metastases. When treated with *Andrographis paniculata* and its compounds alone, twelve patients recovered. All the other patients were treated with standard drugs in addition to the herb; there was no tumor regrowth in forty-seven of these patients within the observational period. Among the twelve patients who recovered using the herb alone, four became pregnant. This is significant because we know that at high doses in animals, *Andrographis paniculata* can have antifertility effects.

With such evidence in hand, American investigators were eager to obtain investigational new drug status from the FDA for an *Andrographis paniculata* extract. In 1996, experiments using the dietary supplement andrographis were conducted to assess safety and dosing of the extract. Early uncontrolled trials demonstrated that the extract safely and effectively blocks growth of both prostate and breast cancer, as well as non-Hodgkin's lymphomas.

After a month or more taking andrographis supplements, six of seven patients exhibited a strong positive response. At the end of the trial, the researchers concluded there had been an incredible 74 percent positive response rate — almost eight out of every ten patients had experienced some tumor shrinkage. This response was measured by traditional clinical variables such as tumor shrinkage for the lymphomas and measures of tumor markers in the blood of individuals with breast cancer. These results are even more impressive when one considers that all the test subjects had undergone chemotherapy without success. Researchers were surprised to discover an unexpected and beneficial psychological side effect in addition to the concrete medical benefits.

The subjects kept journals detailing their experiences. In each case, the journals revealed that the test substance had a positive impact on quality of life. Feelings of well-being increased and there was even an anti-depressant effect. After about four days of treatment, patients were writing that they had an increased feeling of well-being. This side effect cannot be taken lightly; it might help to eliminate the need for antidepressants to help cancer patients cope with the psychological effects of their illness.

Clinical observations of the effects of the andrographis extract dietary supplement was made with nine people. All of them were under the care of a physician and elected to try the supplement without any guarantee of benefit. Results obtained in the ninety-day observation period revealed that the extract was well tolerated. In addition, 80 percent of the individuals reported an increased sense of well-being. Five elected to continue taking andrographis and continued to claim beneficial effects.

Fighting Prostate Cancer

Each year, roughly 317,000 cases of prostate cancer are diagnosed. More American men have prostate cancer than any other form of cancer. With a yearly death rate of forty-one thousand, prostate cancer is the second leading cause of cancer death in the United States. (The first is lung cancer.)

Alarmingly, recent statistics indicate that the age distribution of the disease may be shifting. In 1992, 18.9 percent of those with the disease were eighty or older; in 1996, 13.5 percent were in this age group. Whether men are developing the disease at an earlier age or whether the numbers reflect early diagnosis is unknown. For a man of any age, surgery to remove the prostate is the most common treatment.

Despite the fact that surgical treatment all too often leads to incontinence and/or sexual impotence, the numbers of those opting for surgery more than doubled, from 11.4 percent between 1968 and 1987 to 29.1 percent in 1992. Those in the prime of their lives — patients aged 50 to 59 — were most likely to undergo prostatectomy, surgical removal of the prostate. Extracts from *Andrographis paniculata* promise to offer patients a new treatment option that has no negative side effects.

Initial in vitro testing of andrographis demonstrated that the andrographolide extract is effective in blocking the secretion of a prostate-specific antigen (PSA). A protein released by the prostate gland, PSA increases when cells from the gland become cancerous. Laboratory tests that reveal high levels of PSA are commonly used to diagnose prostate cancer. A normal PSA is 3.99; it is estimated that 90 percent of those whose PSA is 10 or higher will develop cancer. PSA levels are also used to monitor the effectiveness of anticancer treatments.

Studies at the Virginia Prostate Center, which is co-sponsored by the

Eastern Virginia Medical School and the Sentara Cancer Institute, confirm that an extract of *Andrographis paniculata* effectively reduces the level of PSA secreted in prostrate cancer. Studies at the center also showed that an extract of the herb slows the growth of prostate-cancer cells. Furthermore, in tests conducted at the Roswell Park Cancer Institute in Buffalo, New York, the herbal extract was found to have an antiprostate-tumor effect comparable to that of the widely used and highly toxic chemotherapeutic agent cisplatin. Crude extracts of the herb have also been shown to have median effective doses that compare favorably to the median effective doses for the positive control drugs Taxol and etoposide.

Cancer Research and the Plant World

The plant world is no stranger to cancer research. *Andrographis paniculata* is being used as a prime example of the miracles of herbs, but it is just one in a long line of plants being investigated for cancer-fighting properties. Over the past several years, hundreds of plant extracts have been evaluated for their role in preventing cancer. Scientific journals abound with evidence that phytochemicals, chemicals that are found in plants, have many beneficial effects in humans and animals, including the ability to prevent and perhaps treat cancer.

Thanks to the media, we are all, no doubt, aware that vegetables are rich in antioxidants, natural substances that can help prevent the formation of free radicals. Many of us are, however, not sure what free radicals do. These atoms have at least one electron that has no partner. This unpaired electron is highly reactive. In every atom, electrons orbit the nucleus. Because their negative charge balances the positive charge of the nucleus, the overall charge of an atom is zero. When high energy from such sources as light, radiation, or alcohol strikes an atom, an electron is kicked out of orbit. This free-floating electron has absorbed all the energy and is very excited and unstable. It soon links up with another atom to which it transfers its energy. This energized atom, with its extra electron, is a free radical. To return to a stable state, a free radical must transfer its energy to nearby substances.

In the body, free radicals frequently transfer their energy to the fats found in cell membranes, disrupting the membrane and contributing to the development of cancer and other diseases. When free radicals transfer energy to the nucleus and DNA, they can be damged enough to cause malignant changes.

Antioxidants prevent oxidation, the process by which oxygen reacts with another chemical. In doing so, they prevent the damage caused when high energy oxygen produces free radicals. Within the body are natural defense mechanisms that normally prevent such damage. There is, for instance, a protective protein coat that lines the cell membrane, preventing oxygen from reacting directly with the lipids in the cell membrane. Lipids are organic water-insoluble fats, oils, sterols, and triglycerides that, along with proteins and carbohydrates, are the principal structural material of living cells. When oxygen frees its stored energy by reacting with lipids, hydroperoxides may be produced. This, too, can cause the tissue damage that leads to disease.

Antioxidants protect normal cells by warding off the formation of free radicals and the oxidation caused by them. They include a number of vitamins and minerals that are found in plants. The vegetables that have scored highest in antioxidant content are beets, broccoli florets, brussels sprouts, corn, kale, potatoes, red bell peppers, soy, spinach, and sweet potatoes. In addition, chemical compounds called triterpenoids are found in licorice and have been shown to slow rapid division of cells. Other chemicals called terpenes are found in citrus fruit and are known to increase the enzymes that break down carcinogens in the body.

Mounting evidence indicates that consumption of isoflavones, natural estrogens of plant origin, may help to prevent cancer, promote cardiovascular health, and assist in the prevention of joint and bone disease. Isoflavones are found in abundance in soy, a staple of the Japanese diet.

Lessons From Soy and Cancer

In his book *Soya for Health,* Dr. Stephen Holt traces the important effects of soy, particularly soy isoflavones, on cancer. In their classic book *The Simple Soybean and Your Health,* Mark and Virginia Messina state, "...soyfoods are rich in anticarcinogens, substances that, in some way, prevent or control cancer." These scientists drew attention to a milestone in the recognition of the anticarcinogen content of soy foods by discussing the symposium held by the National Cancer Institute in Washington, D.C., in 1990, at which soybeans were described as having at least five individual anticarcinogens.

Furthermore, a recent international symposium on the role of soy in preventing and treating chronic disease provided overwhelming evidence of potential promise for the anticancer effects of soy. The potential anticarcinogenic principles in soy have been listed as protease inhibitors, phytates, phytoesterols, saponins, phenolic acids, and isoflavones.

Protease inhibitors are substances that can block certain enzymes. These inhibitors are ubiquitous in foodstuffs, including soybeans, eggs, cereals, and tuberous legumes. In recent studies, it was demonstrated that breast, skin, and bladder cancer growth was significantly inhibited by soybean diets. Other laboratory studies have confirmed these findings by noting the inhibition of cancers of the lung, colon, pancreas, esophagus, and oral cavity. The mechanism by which protease inhibitors exhibit these beneficial effects in cancer remains poorly understood. Protease inhibitors are, however, known to protect against the damaging effects of radiation and free radicals. Although protease inhibitors are partially destroyed in certain types of food processing, the amount of these substances required to prevent cancer may be quite small. People who ingest sufficient protease inhibitors to prevent cancer would suffer no adverse effects.

Compounds called phytates are abundant in soybeans and other foods that are high in fiber. Phytates may protect against colon or breast cancer, perhaps by blocking iron absorption in the small bowel. Iron is a free radical generator, and free radicals are oxidants that can damage DNA. This damage is regarded as an important preliminary step in cancer promotion. Scientific data reveals that phytates fulfill an antioxidant role similar to that of beta-carotene and vitamin C. Phytates may also be immune stimulators, especially by enhancing natural killer cell function, and phytates could play a role in controlling the growth of cancer cells.

Saponins are a class of glycosides, compounds that have important regulatory, protective, and sanitary functions in plants. Many compounds in this group have physiological effects on humans. Saponins, contained in a variety of plants including soybeans, are believed to play a role in cancer prevention. Evidence points to saponins' antioxidant properties, their ability to prevent mutations, and a possible direct antitumor effect. One study documents an interesting effect of saponins on HIV. This finding is relevant to the anticancer effect since HIV is associated with cancer formation.

Phytoesterols are chemical compounds that may exert a beneficial effect on colon cancer by protecting the colonic mucosa against bile acids and their related metabolic products, which may be carcinogenic. Biliary secretions can enter the colon and be metabolized by certain bacteria to form cancer-promoting compounds. Soybeans also contain phenolic acids, which are antioxidants, and lecithin, which may protect against lung cancer in animals.

The isoflavone content of soy foods presents the most impressive cancer prevention, control, or treatment option. Isoflavones are a group of biologically active compounds that comprise a category of a larger class of compounds known as phytoestrogens. These are compounds of plant origin that have effects similar to the female hormone estrogen, which has several important functions in females. Estrogen stimulates development of secondary sex characteristics as well as growth and maturation of long bones. The hormone also initiates that phase of the sexual cycle (estrus) in which the female is most willing to accept the male.

The chemical structure of isoflavones is similar to that of naturally occurring estrogens, but one hundred times more isoflavone is required to achieve the same effect. Overall, isoflavones affect estrogen levels by functioning as antiestrogens — by binding estrogen receptors and making them available for interaction with more potent, natural estrogens. For example, several types of cancer have estrogen receptors. If an isoflavone attaches to one of these receptors, it can block the more powerful effect of a potent natural estrogen. Through this mechanism of receptor binding, isoflavones and related compounds reduce the sum total of estrogen's effects on tissues and effectively function as partial or complete antagonists of estrogen's effects (i.e., stimulation of long bone development, estrus, and development of breasts). These effects can often be shown to be cancer promoting.

Estrogen receptor stimulation may play a role in the promotion of a variety of cancers, especially breast cancer. In *Preventing Breast Cancer, the Politics of an Epidemic*, Dr. Cathy Read states, "The scientific evidence suggests the protective effect of a diet high in soya proteins may at least partly explain the low rates of breast cancer in China and Japan. The support for the belief that soy-based diets prevent breast cancer (and other cancers, especially prostatic cancer) comes from population studies, the recognition of the 'weak estrogenic effects' of soya isoflavones (genistein and daidzein) and the demonstration of the antiangiogenic effects of genistein." Furthermore, unequivocal anticancer effects of isoflavones have been reported in prostate, colon, and skin cancer.

Many scientists have recently proposed that soy isoflavones may be very important in the prevention and possible treatment of breast and prostate cancer. Soy isoflavones have been proposed as a potential alternative to the use of synthetic or animal derived hormones (Premarin) as hormone replacement therapy. The natural compounds have been shown to suppress menopausal symptoms in double-blind controlled clinical trials in humans, and they are believed to be beneficial in the prevention of osteoporosis, cardiovascular disease, and perhaps age-related cancer that may affect the postmenopausal female.

Dietary supplements composed of soy isoflavones are a convenient way of supplementing a Western diet with this specific health-giving fraction of soybeans. Total isoflavone intakes of up to 120 mg per day appear to be quite safe in adults because these are the amounts of isoflavones that are consumed in soy-based diets. Such diets are common in rural areas in Southeast Asia and are known to be safe and healthful.

Mark and Virginia Messina refer to more than thirty epidemiological studies that have examined the relationship between various types of soy diets and different types of cancer. In a review of these studies, it was concluded that individuals who frequently consume soy foods may have a 50 percent lower risk for many types of cancer than those who do not consume them. The most notable beneficial effects of these foods have been observed in the potential prevention of colorectal cancer, breast cancer, prostate cancer, lung cancer, and gastric cancer. Several studies characterize the beneficial effects of soy diets in the prevention of stomach cancer.

Although the antiestrogenic effects of isoflavones are an important component of the mechanism of their action against cancer, isoflavones possess other beneficial properties that have been the subject of intense research and clinical investigation. Isoflavones are a member of the group of compounds called flavonoids, which are recognized as having anti-inflammatory, antiallergic, antiviral, anticarcinogenic, antineoplastic, antimicrobial, antihelminthic, liver protective, antithrombotic, and antihormonal effects. They act as potent antioxidants, free radical scavengers, and heavy metal chelators — substances that can remove heavy metals from participation in biochemical reactions.

Flavonoids chelate iron and copper, which are oxidant-inducing metals. They facilitate vitamin C stabilization and antioxidant-dependent vitamin C–sparing activities, and enhance vitamin C absorption. Flavonoids have significant effects on enzyme systems that play a role in the development of many chronic diseases, including cancer, arthritis, heart disease, and other inflammatory or degenerative diseases.

Isoflavones are easily utilized by the human body. When taken orally as a food or dietary supplement, they gain access to the systemic circulation and body tissues. The principal isoflavones found in soy include genistein, daidzein, and glycitein. When purchasing dietary supplements, look for these ingredients on the labels.

Researchers have been looking for other chemicals that can mobilize enzymes that aid cells in guarding against such biochemical damage as mutations. Called phase two detoxification enzymes, these include the potent sulforaphane, a phytochemical that appears to make broccoli an excellent cancer fighter. In September 1997, researchers at the Johns Hopkins Medical Institutions in Baltimore, Maryland, found that very young sprouts from broccoli seeds contain twenty to fifty times as many of these chemicals as does mature broccoli.

Investigators have also been looking for phytochemicals that can inhibit cyclooxygenase, which catalyzes the conversion of substances that can stimulate tumor growth, suppress immune surveillance, and activate carcinogens that can damage genetic material. An extract derived from *Cassia quinquangulata* Rich. (*Leguminosae*) collected in Peru was identified as a potent cyclooxygenase inhibitor. It was subsequently found that resveratrol is the active principle in this herb. Resveratrol is a fairly ubiquitous phytochemical found in seventy-two plant species, including grapes, mulberries, and peanuts. It acts as an antioxidant and inhibits tumor development.

Green Tea

In Japan, green tea is recognized as a cancer preventive agent in the diet. Its ability to prevent cancer is so impressive that news of its benefit is beginning to spread to health care givers in Western countries. Both black and green tea are derived from the plant *Camellia sinensis,* but black tea is prepared by fermentation.

Although green tea has known cancer preventive effects, black tea may increase the risk of certain cancers, perhaps due to its content of tannins. The reasons for these different effects on cancer are not entirely clear. It appears that the fermentation of black tea may destroy certain chemicals (polyphenols) found in green tea that have demonstrable antioxidant and cancer preventive effects.

Researchers believe that a substance known as EGCg, a condensed tannin or catechin, gives green tea its anticancer properties. Catechins are present in many different types of tea, but it is EGCg (epigallocatechin gallate) — a powerful antioxidant — that appears to be relatively specific as an anticancer agent in humans and animals.

Most of the early research on green tea's role as a cancer protective agent was performed in Japan by Hirota Fujiki, M.D., and his colleagues. Subsequent animal studies by several groups of researchers throughout the world confirmed these effects. At the M. D. Anderson Cancer Center in Houston, Texas, green tea is being investigated as a source of chemicals that can protect against cancer. In August 1997, the tea entered a phase one clinical trial in the United States.

Dr. Fujiki and his colleagues first reported that the application of EGCg, derived from green tea, inhibited the growth of skin cancer that had been induced in mice through the topical application of a cancer-causing substance. Similar results of the inhibition of cancer growth in animals have been obtained with powdered green tea. Over the past decade, many studies have shown that EGCg and extracts of green tea added to the diet of rats can inhibit the growth of tumors in several organs, including the stomach, duodenum, colon, lung, and pancreas. (For technical details of experiments, see Appendix A.)

K. Imai, M.D., and his colleagues performed a very important study involving 8,552 Japanese in Yoshimi, Japan. Results of the study investigating the potential cancer preventive effects of drinking green tea were presented in part by Dr. Fujiki at the Second Annual Meeting of the Korean Association of Cancer Prevention, which was combined with the Second Interventional Symposium on Cancer Prevention in Seoul, Korea, on November 22, 1997.

Dr. Fujiki explained that the effect of green tea consumption on the occurrence of cancer, cardiovascular disease, and liver disease was studied over a ten-year period, beginning in 1986. The population sample included 419 cancer patients (244 males and 175 females). The individuals with cancer were questioned regarding the quantity and frequency of green tea consumption. The data were adjusted for smoking habits, alcohol consumption, and diet. The relative risks of developing common cancers such as lung, colon, liver, and stomach cancer were calculated to be lower in those who consumed more than ten cups of green tea per day. Furthermore, green tea appeared to delay the onset of several types of cancer.

Certainly, herbs' ability to prevent or treat cancer would be a boon to mankind. Herbs may also provide new ways to diagnose cancer.

Creating New Diagnostic Tools

In addition to developing therapies, signal transduction technology can help in the development of products for the early diagnosis of cancer. Such products also will enable physicians to determine the duration of any remission period.

One of the earliest indications that a normal cell is undergoing transformation to a cancer cell is the presence of the enzyme known as CDK-1. Tests that reveal this enzyme's presence in tissue samples can be used to detect chemically induced cancer in laboratory rodents.

Another enzyme called CDK-2 can also be used in the diagnosis of cancer. The role of CDK-2 in cell division is known; it is also known that this protein is elevated in cancerous cell lines and tumors. Therefore, CDK-2 is an ideal diagnostic indicator for a large number of cancers. As a very early indicator of cell transformation, CDK-2 levels can provide physicians with a greater range of therapeutic options. It is currently being used in the diagnosis of prostate cancer in humans as well as in diagnosing canine bone, lung, and blood cancers.

In individuals with benign prostate hyperplasia (abnormal increase in size of the organ), CDK-2 can be used to identify men who may be at high risk for developing metastatic prostate cancer. Males with metastatic prostate cancer have four times more CDK-2 in their serum than healthy males. CDK-2 can also be used to monitor for recurrence of cancer after treatment.

One drawback to CDK-2 testing is that it cannot be used to ascertain precisely where a cancer is located. This problem can easily be bypassed by using a panel of cancer biomarkers. If, for instance, a physician suspected prostate cancer, he could use prostatic acid phosphate, prostate-specific antigen, *and* CDK-2 to confirm his suspicions.

In veterinary medicine, early diagnosis of cancer in dogs and cats has been limited by the expense of using a number of tissue-specific tumor biomarkers. Now, veterinarians can check an animal's serum for CDK-2, which would result from any tumor tissue. A single test to determine CDK-2 levels can be a cost-effective part of routine dog and cat physicals.

Assessing Carcinogenic Risks

The ability to recognize that a cell is becoming cancerous enables scientists to assess and, hopefully, control carcinogenic risks. New discoveries in cell cycle regulation and cell proliferation offer a new model of chemical carcinogenesis and an improved method of estimating the risk of exposure.

To learn exactly how control of cell division becomes unregulated, many investigators are studying the effects carcinogens have on the cell cycle. Because increased activity of CDK-1 is, for instance, seen in a very large number of cancers, increased levels of the enzyme may signal cells to divide and multiply. Increased CDK-1 levels may be an indicator of carcinogenic potency.

Evidence supporting the relationship between aberrant CDK activity and cancer continues to mount. In addition, CDKs' central role in cell cycle control suggests that chemically induced CDK-1 activity and other cell cycle regulatory proteins may be a critical factor in carcinogenesis induced by chronic chemical exposure.

Some carcinogens do not damage DNA; they are referred to as nongenotoxic. These carcinogens may produce excessive cellular proliferation of one particular tissue, resulting in a high rate of DNA synthesis. The high rate of DNA replication carries an inherent number of genetic errors that may facilitate the formation of tumors. When studying liver cancer, researchers found that many nongenotoxic liver carcinogens do not maintain elevated rates of DNA synthesis with chronic exposure, but tumors still develop. The expression of cell cycle control proteins may provide new ways of assessing risk involved in nongenotoxic carcinogens.

Because nongenotoxic liver carcinogens induce cellular proliferation, studies may elucidate the specific signal transduction pathways stimulated by these carcinogens.

TCDD is one substance that is carcinogenic to the liver. This carcinogen is a dioxin, one of several carcinogenic hydrocarbons that occur as impurities in herbicides derived from petroleum. TCDD causes severe weight loss, a wasting away of the thymus gland, damage to the liver, fetal malformations, and interference in the regulation of both cellular differentiation and proliferation in mammals. Although the extent of the distribution and human exposure are largely unknown, TCDD may pose a threat to humans because it is widespread in landfills, industrial accidents, and herbicides.

Before signal transduction technology, little was known about the molecular basis of TCDD toxicity. Even more troublesome was the lack of any sensitive indicator for assessing biological systems' exposure to TCDD. Scientists now know TCDD's effect on signaling pathways and cell cycle control enzymes. Signal transduction technology has provided an explanation for the variety of biological effects observed when biological systems are exposed to the toxin.

Studies imply that increases in the activity of specific membrane proteins and subsequent alterations in signal transduction play a role in producing the characteristic toxic manifestations of TCDD. Following signal transduction studies, researchers concluded that TCDD can act as a tumor promoter by modulating certain signaling pathways that control the proliferation program of cells.

In one study, dose-related increases of positive cell cycle regulators were noted. During the five days of the study, TCDD dosing resulted in increased activity of the tumor suppressor proteins p53 and Rb and three CDK inhibitory proteins. (See Appendix A for additional information.)

This new understanding should help us test for exposure to chemical carcinogens. With the ability to recognize exposure comes the ability to withdraw the toxin. When the exposure is terminated, proliferative signals cease, which results in the death of excess cells and a return to the cell cycle's resting state.

Thanks to signal transduction technology, scientists have an excellent understanding of liver carcinogenesis. They know, for instance, that induction of cellular proliferation and inhibition of the cell cycle at one identified stage is associated with most tumor promoters. At this stage, the inhibition of communication within the liver has been observed after five weeks of chronic exposure to such toxins as phenobarbital and polychlorinated biphenyls.

It is now possible to create a general model of liver carcinogenesis resulting from chemical toxins. The model shows a cascade of proliferative signaling characterized by increases in CDK-1 activity, increases in DNA synthesis as early as twenty-four hours after dosing, and activation of certain enzymes (tyrosine kinase). This kind of cell signalling involves a message to divide and multiply that results in the increased levels of certain enzymes that are very important to the occurrence and survival of cancer cells. Increased CDK-1 activity is the agent of signal transmission for action in the cell. Replication of DNA occurs in rapidly dividing cells, be they normal or cancerous.

Data suggest that after exposure, cells enter a period of "conflict" between proliferative stimuli and signals to arrest the cell cycle. DNA comprises the storehouse of genetic information in the cell referred to as the genome. DNA damage may result from early rounds of induced cellular division or oxidative damage. Thus, genomic (DNA) instability may occur, resulting in cellular transformation. Armed with this model, researchers should soon find a way of aborting the signals that lead to liver cancer.

Conclusion

There are, no doubt, those who are skeptical about the role of *Andrographis paniculata* and other herbals in effectively treating cancer. Some of the doubts arise because early evidence comes from China, Thailand, and India. We do not think of these countries in terms of scientific accomplishments, technological marvels, or medical breakthroughs. Many people would be more impressed by the evidence if the research were being done in America.

American scientists — like American physicians — find the words *natural, herbal,* or *botanical* equal to *superstition, fad,* or *magic.* The use of natural materials is simply outside their frame of reference.

Natural pharmaceuticals have been held in low esteem in America, and few members of the scientific establishment have been willing to look "backwards" at herbs. In refusing to reinvent the wheel, so to speak, some scientists have instead created a vicious cycle: If countries are not hotbeds of technological marvels, then the scientific establishment will not seriously consider their herbal medicines nor their research — even when double-blind and controlled. If, in addition, American scientists refuse to investigate herbal medicines, how are they to discover whether they are medical marvels? Parochial basis in medicine does not lead to treatment breakthroughs.

The cancer statistics are too frightening for us to ignore any possible treatment. The statistics are most frightening in developing countries where the death rate from cancer is 50 percent higher than in industrialized nations. Throughout the world, the need for treatments that are safe, effective, and accessible is obvious. Herbal-based treatment will fulfill these needs. In the third world, herbal treatments will be especially amenable to people who have long depended on nature, and unlike synthetic drugs, herbals are affordable. As an extra bonus, herbal treatments will provide citizens of developing countries with work harvesting and processing.

When herbal medicine and modern technology meet, the barriers to our understanding and acceptance of nutriceuticals collapse. Signal transduction technology and other biotechnology research should help take us back to the beginnings of medicine, reinvent pharmaceuticals, and bring cancer sufferers real hope.

8

Bringing the Revolution
to Heart Disease

A pear-shaped muscle the size of your fist separates life from death. Inside your chest, protected by your rib cage, your heart muscle beats an average of 103,680 times each day, and each day, your beating heart pumps 2,500 gallons of blood around your body. If your heart stops beating, if the blood stops pumping, your World—your life—will probably come to an end.

Since it's such a small organ and has such a vitally important job, it's no wonder witch doctors and surgeons alike shrank from it in awe. Although primitive witch doctors drilled holes in people's skulls, no one considered operating on a human heart until the twentieth century. Until then, physicians had considered heart surgery the ultimate risk.

In 1944, soldiers in World War II were dying of chest wounds by the score. Then, in June of that year, an army surgeon named Dwight Harken removed a large foreign body from a soldier's right ventricle. So began a road that led eventually to the first successful heart transplant, performed by Christiaan Barnard, M.D., in Cape Town, South Africa, in 1967.

Along the way, improved surgical procedures have led to the replacement of heart valves and vein grafts. Since 1964, the technique of angioplasty has been used to treat occluded or blocked vessels (primarily arteries). During this procedure, a balloon is inserted into an artery narrowed by fatty deposits and is then inflated to clear away the deposits, widen the artery, and improve blood flow.

In 1967, surgeons at the Cleveland Clinic developed bypass surgery for the treatment of coronary obstructions. In bypass surgery, a new vessel replaces one that is obstructed. The new vessel can be synthetic (Dacron), a vein from another part of the patient's own body, or a vein from an animal, usually a pig.

Surgery Isn't a Cure-All

Today, angioplasty and bypass surgery are routine. Approximately 800,000 such procedures are performed in the United States each year, but the operations are not a cure-all.

Dilation of the vessel is achieved in only 90 percent of angioplasty procedures. In 4 to 5 percent of these cases, the procedure fails and emergency replacement of the vessel is required. If the procedure is a failure, there is a 5 percent mortality rate. Also, angioplasty is not considered a "durable" treatment; restricted blood flow recurs in 30 percent of patients within six months; 50 percent of the patients will ultimately require a repeat procedure. Patients who experience retinosis — an overall decrease in the diameter of the treated blood vessel — often undergo angioplasty a second time. When the procedure is repeated, there is a 30 percent chance that an area of tissue will die due to an obstructed blood supply.

As the result of a natural physiological process, the diameter of the treated blood vessel decreases after angioplasty. During angioplasty, a layer of cells lining the vessel (endothelial cells) can be rubbed off. These cells normally prevent platelets (the particles in blood plasma that promote clotting) from sticking to the artery wall. When the cells have been scraped off, platelets can adhere to the arterial walls. Endothelial cells also produce substances that dilate vessels by relaxing smooth-muscle cells, and hinder the growth factors that stimulate cell proliferation. After surgery, the injured smooth-muscle cells multiply unchecked. Eventually, these cells will help to clog the vessels.

Cardiac specialists often advocate angioplasty in the hope that it will eliminate the need for open-chest coronary bypass surgery, a more extensive procedure. Many patients who have angioplasty, however, eventually require coronary artery bypass grafts. Although the operations may be technically successful, patients achieve successful outcomes with the grafts in only 50 to 65 percent of the cases — and the procedure is not without risks.

It has been shown that antioxidants within the body are depleted during aortic coronary artery surgery. This occurs because of the stress of clamping the aorta. Postoperative fever is very common in the first twenty-four hours, and the overall postoperative mortality rate is 1 to 2 percent. In 1 to 30 percent of cases, kidney failure can occur. If the failure is severe enough to require dialysis, the mortality rate is as high as 80 percent. Myocardial infarction (death of an area of heart muscle due to interrupted blood supply) occurs in another 20 to 50 percent of angioplasty cases. Transient neurological deficiencies and postoperative psychosis syndrome have also been seen.

Like angioplasty, coronary artery bypass grafts are not permanent. The veins grafted to detour around blocked arteries are not expected to last more than seven to ten years. Surgeons would like to extend the life of these veins, but they cannot use synthetic substitutes. Because platelets stick to anything man-made, blood clots may form in synthetic vessels that will then become occluded.

Coronary artery bypass grafting is still considered superior to other medical treatments in long-term relief of angina (spasmodic attacks of suffocating chest pain), and in improving functional capacity. However, there is no difference in rates of myocardial infarction between patients who have had the surgery and those who have been medically treated.

Clot-dissolving drugs used in the emergency treatment of heart attacks appear to be as effective as angioplasty. In a study reported in the *New England Journal of Medicine* in June 1997, 10 percent of angioplasty patients died or had heart attacks or strokes within one month of the procedure, while 14 percent of patients receiving clot-busting drugs had similar episodes in the one-month period. After six months, no differences were seen. Furthermore, drugs that dissolve clots, known as thrombolytic agents, also help to save those with blood clots in their lungs.

German researchers have found that patients with clots in the lung, or the main artery in the lung, live longer and are less likely to get new clots when they are treated with clot-busters. One study of 719 patients with clots compared 169 who received clot-busters with 550 who did not. After 30 days, 11.1 percent of those who had not received the clot-busters died, while only 4.7 percent of those who had received the clot-busters died.

In *The Textbook of Surgery*, Gregory L. Moneta, M.D., and John M. Porter, M.D., of the Oregon Health Sciences University, wrote, "Vascular surgeons appear to be approaching the limits of technical competence." The physician-authors go on to say that the field requires "improved understanding and ultimate modifications" of the processes involved in the thickening and hardening of arterial walls due to cholesterol and fat deposits (atherosclerosis), the development of blood clots, and the healing of injured arteries. Researchers are attempting to achieve these goals.

Understanding Hemostasis

Researchers have yet to fully understand hemostasis — the way in which the body curtails bleeding. While clot production is necessary to healing, clotting control is necessary to preserve circulation. Scientists already know that platelets found in the blood plasma of mammals collect during the process of clotting. The platelets adhere to exposed collagen — the protein in connective tissue — and interact with signals released by injured vascular endothelium. In order for an injured blood vessel to stop bleeding, vascular, platelet, and plasma activity must be counterbalanced by mechanisms that limit the accumulation of platelets in the area of injury.

Hemostasis also depends on the formation of a fibrin clot. Fibrin is a protein that forms a fibrous network in the coagulation of blood. This process involves the conversion of inactive substances to their active state through the action of enzymes. When, for instance, platelets are activated, they link and position the clot where it is needed. Free-floating or unnecessary fibrin would result in clots that obstruct the flow of blood. The primary mechanism for inhibiting fibrin is dissolution by plasmin. This substance circulates in its inactive form, plasminogen, which is found within each fibrin clot. Proper levels are maintained through feedback loops and crossover effects involving both amplification and inhibition.

Tissue plasminogen activator (TPA) is sometimes used to treat people in the early stages of a heart attack or stroke. Its use can, however, lead to dangerous bleeding within the brain — an intracerebral hemorrhage, which can lead to a stroke. In June 1996, however, TPA was approved by the FDA for use with ischemic strokes. In these cases, which account for 80 percent of strokes, brain tissue dies because the blood supply is cut off by a clot or narrowed blood vessel. In order for treatment to be effective, TPA must be administered within three hours of the onset of stroke. TPA should not be used by people who have suffered a ruptured vessel in the brain.

Signal transduction technology can be used to help investigators understand the process by which platelets clump together. At New York

Medical College in Westchester, New York, for instance, Carolyn J. Smith, Ph.D., obtained an NIH grant to study cell cycle control in vascular injuries.

Basically, Dr. Smith is studying transduction mechanisms responsible for initiating changes in small muscles. Understanding these changes might enable physicians to curtail the vascular blockages caused by the runaway duplication of muscle cells. One substance being studied is an enzyme in smooth muscles that initiates the transfer of certain chemicals. Dr. Smith hypothesizes that this protein targets transcription factors — genes that signal other genes to turn on later. Inhibitors of the enzyme might interfere with the work of the genes and therefore keep the structure of the blood vessels from changing.

Research to understand the signals involved in bleeding and blood vessel development is beginning to bear fruit. In one study, eight individuals received single doses of a dietary supplement in the form of a commercially prepared extract of *Andrographis paniculata*. All the subjects demonstrated a rapid increase in the time it took platelets to clump. Twelve hours after the extract was administered, however, the effect on platelet massing began to decrease.

Furthermore, it appears that signals involved in vascular injury can be altered by an extract of *Andrographis paniculata*. A number of reports have indicated that the extracts can prevent naturally occurring arterial narrowing as well as strictures that occur after angioplasty. Despite the administration of any number of drugs and other interventional maneuvers, the narrowing of blood vessels following surgery remains an unsolved problem. Test results suggest that *Andrographis paniculata* extracts can significantly alleviate the blockage induced by injury to the cells that line blood vessels and by high-cholesterol diets. An extract of *Andrographis paniculata* has also demonstrated the ability to prevent clot formation and protect the heart muscle against damage that occurs as a result of an obstructed blood supply.

It was demonstrated in rabbits that the herbal extract can inhibit the arterial thickening associated with angioplasty. In one study, rabbits received the extract for three days prior to undergoing angioplasty and for four weeks after surgery. The herbal extract was shown to significantly alleviate plaque-related strictures induced by both injury to the blood vessel and cholesterol in the diet. While arterial narrowing occurred in 100 percent of the control animals, only 70 percent of the animals receiving *Andrographis paniculata* showed stricturing.

Four weeks after the angioplasty in the animals, the blood vessels were examined by angiography, x-ray examination following the injection of radio-opaque substances. In the control group that had undergone surgery, angiography revealed that all dilated arteries showed severe narrowing. In the experimental group, arteries that had undergone surgery showed no narrowing or only mild constriction. It appears that doses of the easily prepared, inexpensive, and safe herbal extract may be quite effective in preventing repeated narrowing of vessels after coronary angioplasty. We have seen that postoperative thickening of artery walls is a major drawback of the therapy.

Andrographis paniculata Is Antithrombolytic

Most arterial clots occur in the elderly or seriously ill. These clots are the result of a buildup of fat deposits on the interior walls of arteries, or of chronic degenerative disease in the wall of an artery. Both conditions cause a buildup of plaque that obstructs blood flow. If blood flow is significantly impeded for six to twelve hours, tissue death will occur. Although there are drugs that can treat acute arterial occlusion, they carry the risk of systemic complications, are expensive, and have the potential to cause hemorrhage.

Arterial occlusion can have serious consequences for any number of organs. When the abdominal aorta is occluded, the condition is life threatening, and survival depends on immediately restarting blood flow. Occlusion in the venous system of the liver occurs primarily in young children, one-and-a-half to three years of age. Patients usually recover promptly, but there is a risk of death from acute liver failure. At present, there is no treatment for this condition. Blockage of the central retinal artery produces sudden, painless blindness.

Emboli that lodge in the lower extremities are usually treated surgically. During the procedure, a catheter with a balloon on its end is inserted as far as possible into the occluded vessel, then the surgeon inflates and withdraws the inflated balloon. Complications can include the loosening of plaque — which increases the risk of future occlusions — and perforation of the vessel.

Clots following open heart surgery can lead to neurological symptoms such as impaired speech, mobility, and sensation. If the blood supply is promptly restored, the symptoms disappear. If not, permanent neurological damage will occur. When clotting occurs in the brain, it cannot receive sufficient blood and oxygen. This will, of course, lead to death of brain tissue and impaired function.

The term *stroke* actually pertains to a sudden loss of brain function due to a blockage or rupture in a blood vessel that feeds the brain. The problem with the blood vessel causes a loss of circulation and a lack of oxygen. Hemorrhagic strokes — those caused by ruptures of blood vessels — account for 20 percent of the cases. Strokes caused by obstructed or clogged arteries are called ischemic and account for 80 percent of cases. At least five different processes can account for ischemic stroke:

- atherosclerosis — deposits in the arteries of plaque containing cholesterol and lipids
- embolus — a mass such as a blood clot, foreign body, or air bubble that travels through the bloodstream, eventually obstructing a vessel
- hemorrhage — extremely heavy bleeding
- thrombus — a clot that forms in a blood vessel or in a heart chamber
- vasospasm — the sudden constriction of a blood vessel resulting in restricted blood flow

In atherosclerosis, yellowish plaques of cholesterol, lipids, and cellular debris form. This plaque encourages obstructions, or thrombi — clots that form in a blood vessel or heart chamber. The formation of thrombi accounts for 33 percent of strokes, and emboli for 31 percent.

Blockage that causes insufficient cerebral circulation can be the result of accumulated platelets, fibrin, and cholesterol. In France and Germany, *Ginkgo biloba* extracts are "approved" (registered) for the treatment of cerebral and peripheral vascular insufficiency. These extracts are among the top three most commonly prescribed drugs in both these countries, with annual sales in excess of $500 million. In the United States, *Ginkgo biloba* is only available as a food supplement.

In Russia and Eastern Europe, peppermint derivatives have played a major role in the treatment of cardiovascular disease. Peppermint is effective in this arena because it blocks calcium entry into cells, thereby exerting action on cardiac and smooth-muscle function. This action is similar to that of many widely used cardiovascular prescription medications.

It appears, then, that it is possible to treat or prevent heart disease without surgical intervention or drugs. Consider that although Eskimos eat a great deal of fat and tend to be plump, they do not get heart disease when they subsist on a traditional diet; the fats they consume are almost all from fish. Fish oil is a natural remedy that could do much more for coronary artery disease than surgical interventions.

Today, researchers know that the fatty acid contained in fish oil is unique. Called omega-3 fatty acids, these substances are now considered by many to be essential to the proper functioning of cells. Omega-3s — found in fatty fish such as mackerel, sardines, salmon, and herring — are safe and more effective than drugs in reducing triglyceride levels in blood. Triglycerides, which can be dangerous to arteries, have been reduced by more than 25 percent in people taking 3,000 to 4,000 mg of fish oil. In addition, studies in Europe have shown that omega-3s can prevent the irregular heartbeats that often prove fatal after a heart attack.

Another natural remedy that seems effective in treating heart disease is the herb *Andrographis paniculata*. Investigators working with Petri dishes, animals, and human beings have demonstrated that an extract of this herb can inhibit the massing and sticking of platelets. In other tests, researchers demonstrated that extracts of *Andrographis paniculata* can actually facilitate the breakdown of clots. The researchers concluded that this herb might be beneficial in preventing and treating conditions in which blood clots form in arteries. An herbal treatment for one of the most prevalent and life-threatening conditions known to medicine would certainly be a revolution in health care. (For details of the studies, see Appendix A.)

In 80 to 90 percent of patients with destroyed heart muscle (acute myocardial infarction), clots are found in the heart shortly after the onset of symptoms. When myocardial or heart muscle tissues are deprived of blood supply, and consequently of oxygen, for a significant amount of time, the tissue dies. Therapy consists of nitroglycerin and/or morphine to relax coronary spasm and relieve pain. Other substances, such as atropine, are administered to restore conduction and increase the heart rate; an electronic pacemaker may also be necessary.

Physicians and researchers today believe that the best treatment is to limit the size of the myocardial infarction in order to preserve pump function. The sign of a healthy heart is the amount of blood pumped out with each beat, which is called the ejection fraction. A healthy heart pumps out 50 percent of the blood it contains.

Therapies that increase oxygen to the myocardium or decrease the heart's need for oxygen are being investigated. In addition, physicians seek to restore the open space in the occluded blood vessel with agents that can break up clots in their early stages. There is substantial evidence that if blood flow can be restored within four hours of the onset of muscle death, a significant amount of heart muscle can be saved. In this case, the mortality rate is lowered and the function of the heart's left ventricle is often better. Many medical people believe that both the clots that cause obstructions and the recurring death of the heart muscle can be prevented by platelet-inhibiting drugs. Agents that can dissolve the clot and increase blood flow through the blocked artery are constantly being sought. *Andrographis paniculata* may possibly fill the bill.

In studies conducted at Tongji Medical University in China, researchers demonstrated that *Andrographis paniculata* may decrease the negative effect of oxygen-free radicals. Because of its beneficial effects on the cell membranes of the heart muscle, the herb can improve heart function.

The same research group also demonstrated that in dogs, *Andrographis paniculata* alleviated the damage that occurs to the heart muscle after blood circulation is restored to the muscle. Evidence of the herb's effects were seen on electrocardiagrams (ECGs). (For details of the study, see Appendix A.)

Another Way of Preventing Coronary Disease

High blood pressure — hypertension — a major risk factor for heart attack or stroke, affects about one fourth of the U.S. population. The condition is usually treated with drugs, but this regimen can be difficult to comply with because of its expense and side effects. In a 1988 study of hypertensive patients, researchers found that people frequently stopped taking their blood pressure medications because of negative side effects. Diuretics increase urine discharge, which can reduce pressure within vessels, but diuretics also cause the loss of potassium, magnesium, and calcium, minerals that play a role in *preventing* heart attack. Diuretics also increase the likelihood that platelets will clump and form clots. Therefore, diuretics may actually increase the risk of heart attack and stroke. Beta-blockers defeat the action of a hormone (noradrenaline) that causes the constriction of blood vessels and an increase in heart rate, blood pressure, and blood sugar levels. These drugs also elevate the levels of cholesterol and certain fats found in the blood, possibly clogging arteries. Long-term use can even lead to heart failure.

A controlled study conducted in 1991 involved the combined use of nutrition, hygiene, and drug therapy in the treatment of high blood pressure. A significant proportion of the patients reported an overall worsening of their condition or development of a new condition over the course of twelve months. Patients who did not have very severe disease appeared quite beleaguered by the drug therapy. These findings highlight the need for gentler approaches to treatment.

A number of nonpharmacological strategies can be used to control hypertension. In many cases, blood pressure can be controlled through weight reduction, salt restriction, moderation of alcohol intake, stress management, exercise, and the cessation of smoking. These lifestyle adjustments, however, can be even more difficult for patients than following the drug regimen, and these interventions are sometimes overlooked by practitioners who are geared to using drug therapies. According to the *Journal of the American Medical Association*, "Treatment of hypertension has become the leading reason for visits to physicians as well as for drug prescriptions." Obviously, commercial interests have little to gain from natural or dietary interventions. Antihypertensive therapy is big business: Sales of blood pressure medications are approximately $10 billion each year. Given the expense and side effects of drug therapy, as well as the difficulty of changing one's lifestyle, a nontoxic, inexpensive substance that could naturally lower blood pressure would be ideal.

In 1987, researchers reported that an extract of *Andrographis paniculata* has antihypertensive effects. When the extract was administered intravenously to spontaneously hypertensive rats, blood pressure was lowered. Experiments were conducted using isolated tissue preparations involving the artery connecting the intestine with the abdominal wall (the mesenteric artery). The extract inhibited the increased pressure induced by noradrenaline. Secreted by the brain, this hormone causes the constriction of blood vessels as well as increases in heart rate, blood pressure, and blood sugar levels. The herbal extract also inhibited electrically induced contraction of the main duct through which semen is carried and certain experimentally prepared guinea pig vessels.

Researchers hypothesize that *Andrographis paniculata* has an antihypertensive effect because it relaxes vascular smooth muscle. The herb may interfere with signals in the vascular system, including enzymes that can cause heart muscle contraction, or relaxation in smooth muscle.

Conclusion

Throughout the world — in developing nations as well as in industrialized countries — heart disease and stroke are the two leading causes of death. In 1990, for instance, 6.26 million people in the world died of heart disease and 4.38 million died of stroke. Each year, more than 500,000 deaths in the United States are attributed to heart disease. In 1995, 737,563 Americans were felled by diseases of the heart. In that same year, stroke killed another 157,991.

In the United States, stroke is the third leading cause of death and is the leading cause of long-term disability, the total cost of treatment exceeding $23 billion a year. People who have high blood pressure, heart disease, or a high red-blood cell count are most at risk, and smoking cigarettes increases that risk. Males, African-Americans, and people with a family history of stroke are also at increased risk. Once a person passes the age of 55, risk doubles every ten years, but each year, 28 percent of the victims are under the age of 65.

This year, more than 1,500,000 Americans will have a myocardial infarction; 500,000 of them will die of complications, and approximately 33 percent of patients with coronary disease will experience sudden death without angina or myocardial infarction. It is believed that most of these die as the result of decreased blood supply caused by the constriction or obstruction of blood vessels.

Keeping blood and oxygen flowing to the brain — a job that *Andrographis paniculata* appears capable of accomplishing without side effects or great expense — can save countless lives *and* improve the quality of life for scores more. If the flow of blood to the brain is restricted by clotting or narrowing of vessels, insufficient oxygen and nutrients reach the organ. Diminished blood flow can cause short-term memory loss, ringing in the ears, dizziness, headaches, depression, and impaired mental performance. If the loss of blood is prolonged, brain tissue will die.

The ability to treat or prevent arterial clots with a noninvasive technique is truly a boon to mankind. Since *Andrographis paniculata* is an inexpensive, all natural, nontoxic substance that is readily available, its benefits might help to revolutionize cardiac care. And andrographis is only one of thousands of herbal options — options, which may help in the treatment of cancer, heart disease, and even AIDS.

9

Defeating AIDS With Herbal Miracles

AIDS — the mere sound of the word evokes a shudder, and we are, perhaps, reminded of the diseases that have plagued mankind through the ages. The Old Testament reports plagues in Egypt more than three thousand years ago. Subsequently, the Plague of Justinian — probably bubonic plague — in the sixth century lasted fifty years and wiped out three million people in the Middle East. During the bubonic plague, or Black Death, of the fourteenth century, one-third of Europe's population, almost thirty million people, perished. In the nineteenth century, cholera, flu, and polio epidemics aroused as much terror as the word *Ebola* does today. But AIDS is different from all the rest, transmitted not by rodents or food or air but by the most basic component of human life — bodily fluids.

AIDS — acquired immune deficiency syndrome — is a worldwide problem that appears to have its roots in Africa. Many epidemiologists believe that the AIDS epidemic started when a virus in African primates somehow, probably through mutation, entered the human race. In fact, blood that had been stored in Zaire since 1959 shows some evidence of human immunodeficiency virus (HIV), the cause of AIDS. Many villages in central Africa have literally been decimated by AIDS. It is estimated that 5 percent of the population in Africa is infected with HIV; 60 percent of the world's cases of HIV occur in sub-Saharan Africa.

In an era of easy passage from one part of the world to another, it is not surprising that AIDS soon spread to North America, Asia, and the third world countries. The first North American cases were reported in 1981 when the condition still had no official name. Today, as the result of the investigation of hospital records and tissue samples frozen following a death in 1969, we know that AIDS has been in North America even longer than originally believed. It was not until 1983 that there was concrete scientific evidence that AIDS was caused by the human immunodeficiency virus, or HIV. Today, two strains have been identified; these are known as HIV-1 and HIV-2. AIDS in the United States is caused almost exclusively by HIV-1; HIV-2 seems confined to Africa.

The Nature of the Aids Virus

A virus cannot live on its own or reproduce itself. When a virus finds a suitable body cell, proteins on the outside, or envelope of the virus, attach to receptors on the cell. HIV enters human cells by binding to two molecules on the cell's surface. One of these — CD4 — was identified in 1984. The other, more recently identified molecules, are the coreceptors CCR5 and CXCR4.

HIV cells tend to cluster in the brain and in certain skin tissues, just as the hepatitis viruses cluster in the liver or the cold virus in the nose and throat. HIV is also attracted to helper T cells, which get their name from the thymus glands where they are activated. Helper T cells signal lymph nodes and the spleen to produce more antibodies, chemical weapons that are released into the bloodstream to fight infection. Once the antibodies have conquered the invader, suppressor T cells produce chemicals that signal an end to the production of antibodies until they are needed again.

When the virus attaches to the helper T cell, the envelope opens and the RNA spills out. Then RNA from the virus moves into the cell's nucleus and is transcribed into viral DNA with the aid of an enzyme called reverse transcriptase, which the virus needs to copy its genetic material. The virus then tricks the cell into producing virus chemicals instead of those it usually makes. The T cells, in effect, become virus-producing factories; they no longer function as helper T cells.

DNA in a normal or uninfected cell tells that cell to reproduce and make more helper T cells. DNA in an infected cell sends a signal to make more virus and leave a dead T cell behind. Without T cells, the lymph nodes and spleen never receive signals to fight off invading organisms. When a person develops AIDS, enough T cells are destroyed to seriously damage the immune system. This damage is deadly: Over 60 percent of those diagnosed with AIDS have died. Advances in treatment are beginning to change that statistic, but the risks remain.

The Risk of AIDS Is Real

Once considered a disease of gay males and intravenous drug users, AIDS soon knew no boundaries: Heterosexual males and females became its victims through sexual contacts as well as exposure to tainted blood. These threats are as real today as they were in the 1980s. Although the rate of infection has declined among males over thirty, it has remained relatively constant among women and minorities, and the risk to teenagers is increasing. Today, public health experts believe that condoms provide the best defense against the AIDS epidemic.

We cannot consider ourselves safe when more than forty-three thousand Americans died of HIV infection in 1995, making it the eighth leading cause of death in the United States that year. Just consider that only five years earlier, AIDS had been at the bottom of the list of the thirty most common causes of death worldwide. The Orphan Project in New York City now estimates that by the year 2000, between seventy-two thousand and one hundred and twenty-five thousand children will be motherless as a consequence of AIDS, and the U.S. Census Bureau predicts that by the year 2010, death rates in Haiti and some South African countries will be twice as high as normal—because of AIDS.

Despite the efforts of activist groups, educators, and researchers, the disease continues to spread, though more slowly. The World Health Organization estimates that approximately ten million people are now infected by the HIV virus. The epidemic has already killed more than 4.5 million worldwide and is growing by more than three million cases a year. It is believed that every American knows at least one person who has died of AIDS. Yet, some experts believe that the AIDS risk is actually increasing because we are becoming complacent about the disease, believing that the risks are limited to intravenous drug addicts and the promiscuous. Some people have been lured into a false sense of security, vainly trusting that AIDS drugs can cure them if they do get the disease.

Abstinence and safe sex dramatically reduce your risk, but there are other possible sources of infection that are more difficult to control. The risk of receiving contaminated blood—though slight—is real. It is currently estimated that testing will uncover six hundred tainted units of blood out of the twelve million units donated each year. More frightening still is the estimate that HIV contamination exists in twenty units that are *not* identified as tainted. Remember, it takes eight to twelve weeks before the virus can be detected in the blood of an exposed individual. If a person donates blood during that time period, the blood will test negative even if it contains the AIDS virus.

The costs in human suffering cannot be measured. We can, however, count the dollar cost: Each case in the United States costs society an average of $100,000. The cost of AIDS reaches millions of dollars when lost productivity is included. Progress in providing a cure has been painstakingly slow. As long as the danger of infection with HIV persists, the need for effective and readily available treatment is paramount.

Drug research has focused on inhibiting viral replication, the action of drugs such as zidovudine (AZT) and Saquinavir. Today, combination drug therapy seems to prolong life and greatly improve the quality of that life. The Panel on Clinical Practices for Treatment of HIV Infection released a statement in June 1997 that says, in part, "Three-drug therapy is the preferred choice, and any drug regimen that does not achieve maximum viral suppression is not optimal."

The combination of drugs is often referred to as a cocktail and consists of synthesized inhibitors of protease and reverse transcriptase. Protease inhibitors block enzymes necessary for replication of the AIDS virus and keep it from assembling new parts. These inhibitors are administered in combination with other agents, such as reverse transcriptase inhibitors, because resistance to any one protease inhibitor occurs within a few weeks. Reverse transcriptase inhibitors such as AZT and 3TC work by disrupting reproduction of the virus.

Cocktail therapy may not be quite as effective as initially supposed, especially in patients with established AIDS. Some statistics, however, indicate that combination therapy reduces viral replication by 99 percent, lowering the mortality rate from 10.1 percent to 5.87 percent. Largely because of these treatments, overall AIDS deaths did not increase in 1996 for the first time since the early 1980s, and from January to September 1996, AIDS deaths actually fell by 19 percent. In September 1997, government agencies announced a 26 percent decrease in AIDS deaths. For the first time in years, AIDS was not the leading cause of death among young men aged twenty-five to forty-four. It had fallen to number two, behind accidents (automobile, sports-related, weapon-related, and so forth).

At the fourth Conference on Retroviruses and Opportunistic Infections held in Washington, D.C., in January 1997, David Ho, head of the Aaron Diamond AIDS Research Center in New York City, advised caution. He declared, "We must paint the situation in the proper shade of gray." Mary Ann Chiasson, assistant commissioner of the New York City Department of Health, reported a drop of 30 percent in AIDS deaths but suggested that the decline might be linked to an increase in federal funding for AIDS patients. Reducing the amount of HIV in the blood doesn't necessarily mean a patient will suffer from fewer AIDS-related diseases. Scientists are not certain how long the new combinations of drugs will work before resistant strains appear. Presenters pointed out that physicians who prescribe single drugs or inadequate doses may inadvertently encourage resistant strains. In addition, protease inhibitors do not work for everyone.

While deaths decreased 28 percent among whites, they fell only 16 percent among Hispanics and only 10 percent among blacks. Some fear that the drugs have made us complacent about the disease. Jeffrey L. Reynolds, director of policy for the Long Island Association for AIDS CARE, Inc., points out that the number of those who become infected each year continues to rise. The number of drug users, women, and teens in particular, is increasing. Reynolds fears that many are abandoning safe sex in the belief that the disease "simply means popping a few pills each day…it would be ironic if medical advances designed to solve a public health crisis actually made it worse, but in some ways that's what seems to be happening."

What many people don't know is that the absorption of protease inhibitors is small so that large doses — thirty-six pills a day — are required. For many, this combination therapy is prohibitively expensive, costing from $8,000 to $16,000 a year. The expense of HIV therapies puts them out of the reach of 90 percent of those who are infected around the world. In the United States, it is estimated that 150,000 people take protease inhibitors, which are sold under brand names such as Invirase, Norvir, Viracept, and Crixivan. These protease inhibitors have been linked to potentially dangerous side effects.

Early in June 1997, the FDA issued warnings to physicians that some patients who were taking protease inhibitors had developed diabetes and hypertension. In some patients who were already suffering from these conditions, the diseases became worse. Of eighty-three AIDS patients with the conditions, twenty-seven required hospitalization, and six of those cases were considered life-threatening.

The use of AZT is also fraught with problems. Although it is one of the few antivirals that can slow the HIV infection, AZT has had limited use due to the high incidence of toxic side effects at therapeutic doses. The side effects include nausea and kidney stones. In some cases, there have been links to diabetes and low levels of glucose in the blood (hypoglycemia). Use of the drug can lead to significant bone marrow depression, resulting in anemia that is severe enough to require blood transfusions.

Use of AZT has also been associated with brain and liver toxicity, loss of speech, headaches, insomnia, rash, and itching. Because of the possibility of esophageal ulcers, patients must take the medication with a significant volume of water and are advised not to lie down for at least an hour. Side effects and expense prevent many patients from using the medication.

Many people are morally outraged at the prohibitive cost of AIDS drugs, and are also dismayed at the slow progress that has been made in finding a cure for AIDS. The public outcry has led to criticism of the Food and Drug Administration and the process of drug approval, as well as a search for alternative means of managing the disease. In a quest for treatments that can be produced quickly, cost less, and have fewer side effects, investigators naturally turned to botanicals. However, alternative therapies for AIDS are perhaps the most sensitive subject for regulatory affairs bureaus.

The Rationale for Investigating Herbals

Scientists know that protease inhibitors help block replication of the AIDS virus. They also know that these inhibitors are abundant in plants. Protease inhibitors were found in soybeans in 1947, and nutritionists have known since the 1970s that rice, corn, beans, wild tomatoes, and other vegetables contain these inhibitors. A number of dietary supplements are now standardized for protease inhibitor content.

Some reverse transcriptase inhibitors, which reverse reproduction of the virus, may also occur in nature. Bioflavonoids are found in plants and function in many ways, including the maintenance of small blood vessel walls in animals. Quercetin, a bioflavonoid found in red apples and red onions, has been shown to act against the viruses that cause AIDS, herpes simplex, and polio. Quercetin is also a potent reverse transcriptase inhibitor at concentrations as low as 2 micrograms per milliliter — that's approximately 50 millionths of an ounce of the drug in an ounce of blood.

Investigators also knew that many herbs had traditionally been used in preparing tonics — invigorating or restorative agents. Reputed to have immune-enhancing functions, these herbs might prove effective in the fight against AIDS. Researchers at the China Academy of Traditional Chinese Medicine in Beijing wrote, "The current study of AIDS...concentrated on the inhibition of HIV, that is, the aspect of expelling the pathogenic factor." The Chinese researchers believed — as had Claude Bernard and Elie Metchnikoff before them (see pages 7–8) — that the virus is the cause of the disease but must express itself "through the human body." Enhancing the body's natural ability to expel the invading organism might aid in curing the disease.

Today's Western researchers may at last be joining those who believe that one of the best ways to deal with the consequences of infections is to enhance the body's own defenses. According to a February 1997 issue of the *Medical Herald*, a monthly newsletter for physicians, AIDS investigators are now "developing immunomodulator drugs to strengthen the body's immune system." Immune enhancement has the added advantage of preventing the spread of infectious diseases.

John Siegfried, M.D., vice president for regulatory and scientific affairs at the Pharmaceutical Research and Manufacturers of America, explains that attention had focused on protease inhibitors because they help to prevent reproduction of the HIV virus. In a 1995 issue of the *Journal of Traditional Chinese Medicine,* Dr. Lu Weibo reported that extracts of several herbs might have inhibitory effects on the replication of HIV-1, one of two identified strains of the AIDS virus. He had investigated twenty-seven traditional Chinese medicinal herbs; *Andrographis paniculata* was one of eleven that inhibited HIV replication.

Long used in traditional Chinese medicine, *Andrographis paniculata* is a medicinal herb that has a history of successful use in the treatment of numerous conditions. The herb has been the subject of a considerable amount of research over the past two decades. Much information has, therefore, become available about its pharmacological composition, safety, efficacy, and mechanisms of action in the body. Now scientists believe that this ancient herb can join with modern technology in the fight against our twentieth-century plague, AIDS.

Technology that can reveal how and when messages are carried to cellular particles in order to "turn on" their functions (signal transduction technology) seemed a natural weapon to bring to the war against AIDS. The disease directly affects the cell cycle: The HIV-1 virus produces a gene product that promotes viral replications through its affects on cell cycle messengers. When the technology was applied to studies of *Andrographis paniculata,* substances that destroyed the virus's communications mechanism were identified. Researchers found that one component of the herb — andrographolide — stops the progress of the disease and can also prevent transmission by modifying cellular signal transduction. Andrographolide probably does this by inhibiting enzymes that facilitate the transfer of phosphates. Progress through the cell cycle is regulated, at least in part, by cycles in which high energy phosphates are created or destroyed. The production of these phosphates is the main source of cellular energy.

When the HIV-1 virus infects certain cells, it causes a change in the cell cycle that results in optimal conditions for replication of the virus. *Andrographis paniculata*'s ability to interfere with key enzymes that determine this viral replication process has been well demonstrated in laboratory experiments. These experiments have now shown that extracts of the herb can inhibit the replication of the HIV-1 virus in human lymphocytes, and they work in a synergistic manner with zidovudine (AZT) to augment inhibition.

The hallmark of HIV-1 infection is that the viral replication cycle occurs during specific phases of the cell cycle. HIV-1 has been shown to alter the regulation of the cell cycle by causing it to stop at a particular, identifiable phase. Progression through a normal cell cycle is controlled by a variety of factors, including several types of cellular proteins and enzymes, known as cyclins and cyclin-dependent kinases (CDKs). These form specific complexes that coordinate the process of cell division and the progression of the normal cell cycle phases. The presence of viral gene products is known to result in excess activity of one or more of these cell-regulating proteins or enzymes. HIV's destructive effects have been associated with enhanced activation of CDK.

A particular CDK — CDK-1 — can be called the central information processing protein because its function involves the coordination of all events relating to cell division. As the cell moves through the cell cycle, information concerning the activities of the cell is sent to CDK-1. As long as these signals indicate proper functioning of the cell, movement through the cycle continues. When there is a viral infection, phosphorylation and abnormal CDK-1 activity will usually occur. In fact, researchers at the National Institutes of Health (NIH) have reported that these conditions are present in immune cells (T cells) infected with the HIV virus.

Agents that can prevent phosphorylation can lessen the severity of AIDS; these agents constitute a new class of antiviral compounds that includes andrographolides. Testing has demonstrated that an extract of *Andrographis paniculata* can, in fact, inhibit CDK-1, which undergoes dramatic increases in concentration and activity in cells infected with HIV.

In addition, an extract of the herb was found to inhibit HIV's toxic effect on cells. Extracts of *Andrographis paniculata* appear to be emerging as ideal adjuncts to existing treatments for AIDS. In laboratory studies, an extract of *Andrographis paniculata* has been shown to inhibit HIV-1 propagation. According to Dr. David I. Cohen of NIH's Laboratory of Tumor Biology, agents in the new class of antivirals "may drastically limit" HIV's ability to replicate and may prevent the virus from killing immune cells. (For more information on the tests, see appendix A.)

Testing conducted at the Frederick Research Center offered further evidence of andrographolide's use as an AIDS therapy. These trials demonstrated that extracts of *Andrographis paniculata* increased common AIDS drugs' (AZT's or zidovudine's) ability to inhibit replication of the virus. During the experiments, the combination of AZT and the herbal extract inhibited replication of the virus more than could be accounted for by the effect of either drug used alone. Combining the therapies also permits lower AZT doses, which can decrease cost of the treatment and may significantly reduce toxic side effects.

Laboratory studies conducted at the Frederick Research Center in association with NIH also indicated that the herbal extract inhibits HIV in infected T cells through an entirely new mechanism of action. Investigators think that the herb may interfere with signals generated by the virus and sent to uninfected immune cells. These signals lead to cell death. Inhibition of these signals is at the heart of the herbal extract's role in halting HIV-1 infection. Some researchers believe that andrographis extracts may also be useful in the battle against other viruses, including the Ebola virus and those associated with herpes, hepatitis, and influenza. (For additional information on the mechanism of action, see Appendix A.)

Lives Are Saved

In the halls of science, theories are often tested in petri dishes or test tubes (in vitro) and then in animals. But it is studies with humans — called "clinical trials" — that ultimately reveal the efficacy of a treatment. The first step on the road to clinical trials is evaluation of a test material's safety.

Toxicity studies of andrographis were initially conducted in rats and rabbits that received one gram (less than ¹/₁₆ of an ounce) of the extract per kilogram (2.2 pounds) of body weight daily for seven days. No changes were observed in body weights, complete blood counts, or microscopic evaluation of tissues from liver, kidneys, and other major organs.

Studies of extracts of *Andrographis paniculata* revealed that it has low toxicity in humans: Evidence of toxicity does not appear suddenly, nor does usage seem to lead to chronic side effects. A long history of the use of andrographis in traditional Chinese medicine and widespread contemporary use of this herbal in Scandinavia without toxicity supports andrographis's safety as a dietary supplement.

Early clinical trials were conducted in Tanzania. Experts in the field of traditional Chinese medicine treated 158 AIDS patients over a period of three years with a combination of traditional herbs. Some positive effects were seen in 39.87 percent of the patients. For instance, symptoms such as diarrhea, anorexia, fever, and weight loss were alleviated in 56.5 percent of the cases, and improvement of immune function was seen in 31.01 percent of the patients. Only thirteen patients died.

Observations of the use of *Andrographis paniculata* extract have been made at Bastyr University in Seattle, Washington, a college of natural medicine (naturopathy). Sixteen male and female HIV-1-positive patients over the age of eighteen elected to use andrographis. Their progress was monitored in a well-conducted and detailed manner. The subjects had CD4 counts ranging from 200 to 703.

By checking the level of CD4 in a person's blood, physicians can monitor the course of the disease. When first infected with HIV, people show no symptoms and their CD4 count is approximately 1,000. (The normal level of CD4, a molecule on the cell's surface to which the AIDS virus attaches, ranges from 435 to 1,700.) When the count falls to between 200 and 400, AIDS symptoms such as lymph node enlargement, night sweats, and weight loss begin to appear. The decreased CD4 count indicates that the immune system has been impaired.

None of the patients had hepatitis or other liver abnormalities. None of the individuals who opted to use the specially prepared andrographis extract wanted to use any antiviral therapy or prophylactic antibiotics during the period of observation. All blood and laboratory testing, as well as administration and cessation of substances, was on a completely voluntary basis.

The individuals received 5 mg (approximately 2 ten-thousandths of an ounce) of andrographolide per kilogram (2.2 pounds) of body weight three times a day for three weeks, followed by 10 mg (approximately 3 ten-thousandths of an ounce) per kilogram of body weight three times a day for three weeks. During the final three weeks of the study, no andrographolide was administered. Blood tests to assess the amount of the virus and number of lymphocyte cells (white cells that play a role in the development of immunity) present were conducted every three weeks. In addition, cholesterol and complete blood cell counts were checked before dosing began and again at weeks one, three, four, six, seven, and nine.

Thirteen of the sixteen subjects who took the dietary supplement were observed for nine or more weeks. One of the subjects withdrew due to a severe allergic reaction; two could not tolerate the bitter taste of the herbal preparation. The other three people took the dietary supplement for six weeks; the supplement was well tolerated and produced a median 38 percent decrease in the amount of HIV-1. Transient elevations in the amount of the virus were seen in two subjects, but at six weeks, their viral load had decreased to the range of the other subjects.

In addition, there was a 31 percent median increase in the number of CD4 cells, receptors for HIV. This count shows evidence of the improved status of the immune system: CD4 cells are no longer binding with the virus. This effect has been noted repeatedly in animals and humans in many studies of andrographis. A very slight increase in the liver enzymes AST and ALT was observed in two subjects, which may indicate that some individuals have a lower tolerance for the herb.

In at least two subjects, the evidence of efficacy was truly astonishing. One subject experienced an *83 percent* decrease in HIV-1 viral load and another exhibited a *90 percent* increase in CD4 cells, cells to which HIV binds, in just six weeks. There was a mean rise of 14 percent in serum cholesterol, which was considered to be a measure of the subjects' overall well-being, and an increase in complete white blood cell counts was noted. When the volunteers discontinued the supplement, the beneficial trends appeared to reverse rapidly. Three weeks after cessation of the dietary supplement, all but one of the individuals had returned to prestudy levels. Not surprisingly, the majority of the individuals wished to continue using the herbal extract.

Data obtained during the nine-week observation period with individuals taking the dietary supplement extract indicates that the extract of *Andrographis paniculata* is safe and well tolerated. In addition, the observations — although not a formal clinical trial — suggest that the extract has positive activity in humans infected with the HIV-1 virus. According to Dr. Cohen, the National Cancer Institute is interested in the herbal extracts because of the documented observations, including the reductions in viral loads and the increases in the subjects' CD4 + cell counts in such a short time.

The apparent beneficial effects of andrographis in AIDS may not be directly related to an herbal affect on the HIV-1 virus. It may be that the extracts disrupt the signal transduction pathways that are affected by the virus. This interpretation is consistent with laboratory studies of andrographis using tests to evaluate signals. Signals involved in cell-to-cell transmission of the virus, viral replication, and destruction of immune system cells also appear to be disrupted by the herb. In brief, *Andrographis paniculata* appears to affect HIV infection in two distinct ways:

It inhibits HIV replication by halting transmission of signals or messages within cells.

It halts destruction of immune cells by interfering with HIV signals that contribute to their destruction.

Andrographis paniculata may also prove to be very effective in preventing the spread of the virus.

Preventing Transmission

Sexual transmission of the AIDS virus to women is fast becoming one of the most significant health issues for women worldwide. In most developing countries, heterosexual transmission is the most common mode of transmission of the HIV-1 virus. A January 1997 study revealed that in Asia, the number of new AIDS cases among gay men had decreased, while it had increased among heterosexual women. HIV-1 is now among the top five causes of death for women in developing countries. The risk of contracting the disease is greater than originally imagined.

The techniques being investigated to inhibit transmission of HIV-1 currently use physical processes to deactivate the virus. One such process involves a substance that changes a virus's surface charge so that it cannot attach to receptors on cell membranes. These substances are not well tolerated by humans. Other agents can be administered to increase the acidity of blood so that the virus cannot thrive, but the human body doesn't react well to the increased acidity. Other techniques being investigated are also irritating to people and difficult to administer. Successful curtailing of the AIDS epidemic requires a substance that can be taken orally or applied topically shortly before or after exposure.

In 1995 in an attempt to get better control of the spread of the disease, the Frederick Research Center evaluated one hundred extracts of traditional Chinese medicines under a contract with the NIH. Thirty-two of these exhibited significant capacity to inhibit sexual transmission of HIV. The extracts disrupted the replication of topical cell-to-cell transmission of the HIV-1 virus sufficiently to inhibit the virus's ability to infect healthy individuals. Twenty herbal extracts demonstrated potency equivalent to the positive control used in the study, dextran sulfate. This chemical is one of the most powerful antimicrobial agents available for use in topical ointments. Seven of the herbs were found to be even more potent than the dextran sulfate. Researchers now hope to develop an effective preventative treatment that does not have the side effects of existing synthetic, antiviral agents.

If a preventative option is based on herbal extracts, it can be inexpensively manufactured in developing countries, where the need is so great. In the United States — through the tolerance of regulatory affairs agencies — these compounds can be brought to market quickly because they can be classified as supplements and will not require the extensive testing needed for approval as a drug. Indeed, extracts of *Andrographis paniculata* are already being sold on the world market. Their use through the centuries documents their low toxicity, as does testing in one of the country's most prestigious laboratories. No individual should purvey *Andrographis paniculata* as an AIDS treatment. In addition, no individual, agency, interest group, or government should interfere with a self-reliant AIDS patient who wishes to try an option in the absence of a cure.

Consumer Access to *Andrographis paniculata*

Investigators in the United States now have useful information concerning dose range and are speedily moving forward with the development of dietary supplement products. Given the expected dose ranges of herbs, it is estimated that the annual cost of using the products will be $1,000, as compared to the $8,000 to $23,000 annual cost of current synthetic drug treatments.

Testing conducted in conjunction with the NIH has centered around extracts of *Andrographis paniculata* called andrographolides. These are now available in several commercial preparations in Scandinavia and the Far East, and should be on the shelves of American health food stores in the dietary supplement section. Many types of andrographis supplements may soon appear, and extracts should guarantee standardized amounts of andrographolide.

In the study conducted in Tanzania with such positive results, HIV patients were using herbs that are available in many herbal shops and health food stores. They are sold under such names as chuanxinlian, serpentine herb, and *Andrographis paniculata*. As with any herbal product, consumers should check the products with knowledgeable health care providers and look for standardized extracts. Consumers should also comparison shop: Read labels carefully and look for products that refer to test results and clinical observations. The authors of this book are not making any treatment recommendations but are merely providing an interpretation of their understanding of recent scientific literature.

Conclusion

Imagine a world in which those afflicted with AIDS can plan for the future with confidence and without bankrupting themselves. Imagine a world in which lovers can be guaranteed protection from HIV infection by using an inexpensive, natural, topically applied preparation. Herbs even older than the concept of plague itself show promise of unlocking the door to this world.

Behind that door, the battle against AIDS may be fought with a combination of therapies that will address all aspects of HIV-1 infection: cell-to-cell transmission, virus replication, and T-cell degeneration. A combination of approaches may be necessary to get around emerging viral resistance to therapeutic regimens and successfully manage the disease. AIDS patients typically exhibit malnutrition and imbalances in blood chemistry that may also inhibit immune function. So, just as experts in traditional Chinese medicine predicted, treatment may also require stimulating the immune system. Extracts of *Andrographis paniculata* and other agents might possibly satisfy these needs.

Thanks to signal transduction technology, investigators have been able to identify various steps in the process whereby HIV kills cells. Use of the technology has also provided a foundation for a totally new generation of natural botanicals that can assist in the fight against AIDS. In brief, andrographolides appear to possess many versatile effects, including:

inhibition of cell-to-cell transmission of the HIV-1 virus
halting of viral replication
inhibition of T-cell destruction
synergistic antiviral activity with AZT

By combining the best of modern technology, ancient medical wisdom, and sound scientific research, people may find effective treatment and a decrease in cases of yet another plague.

10

Herbs Used to Treat Common Ailments

Back when the American colonists were arguing with the Mother Country, a band of angry men threw British tea into Boston Harbor. The British would never have wasted tea like this. Not only did they value it as a beverage, they had already discovered its medicinal value. In fact, the act of defying the British may be seen as an abuse of a botanical remedy.

For almost 250 years, the Boston Tea Party has been seen as a pivotal moment on the road to freedom. Today, there's another revolution brewing in America and, once again, tea — or at least the plants from which it is made — can be seen as a pivotal factor.

As we have seen, dissatisfaction with the practice of medicine in America and Western society is playing a large role in the growth of alternative medicine. One alternative that is rapidly becoming popular is the use of herbal medicines or nutriceuticals. A common way to consume herbs is by drinking herbal tea.

There was a time when every household in the Western world had a garden of medicinal herbs. Every housewife knew which herbs in her garden could be used to treat common ailments. She grew, dried, and stored ginger so that when someone was feeling nauseated, she could brew up a soothing tea. When someone had a sore throat, a housewife would grab a handful of horehound (*Marrubium vulgare*) and mix up a tea that would liquefy mucus and soothe the pain.

Few people today know which herbs are commonly used to treat which disorder. It is not possible to cover all of the potential health benefits or medical applications, past and present, of all herbal or botanical agents in a comprehensive manner. Analyzing the therapeutic benefit of a botanical or herbal preparation is an extremely difficult matter. Attempts to review literature on remedies of natural origin is made difficult by statements of "belief" which are often not supported by well-controlled studies.

Before you begin to shop, you should know that herbs have a vast array of therapeutic properties that are referred to in a highly specialized jargon. You will recognize many of the terms that begin with the prefix *anti* followed by the name of the disease or condition the herb controls (e.g., antirheumatic, antibiotic). Some of the terms may, however, be unfamiliar to you. These are summarized in the following list.

Herbal Jargon Defined

Abortifacients Capable of bringing on a spontaneous abortion. (To be feared and not recommended.)

Alterative An herb that works slowly to alter body chemistry. The effects are not immediately noticeable. Restores health and vital functions by cleansing the blood.

Analeptic Having restorative or stimulating effects.

Analgesic A pain reliever.

Anodyne *See* analgesic.

Anthelminthic Botanicals that rid the body of worms.

Antiarrhythmic Preventing or relieving irregular heart rhythms.

Antiemetic Controls vomiting.

Antihistamine Counteracts histamine production in colds and allergies. Histamines are physiological chemicals that are released from cells in the immune system.

Antiphlogistic Reduces inflammation.

Antipyretic Lowers fevers.

Antiscorbutic Botanicals that fight scurvy (these are high in vitamin C). Although scurvy has not been a problem in the United States in several generations, increasing your daily dose of vitamin C can prevent the gum disease that leads to tooth loss and may lessen your chance of catching a cold.

Antiseptic Prevents infection by inhibiting the growth of micro-organisms.

Antispasmodic Controls muscle spasms.

Aperient Gently stimulates bowel elimination.

Aphrodisiac Arouses or intensifies sexual desire.

Aromatic Substances that contain volatile oils; often spicy smelling; they stimulate digestion.

Astringent These herbs contract tissues; effective in stopping the flow of bodily fluids such as blood.

Bronchodilator Widens air passages; relaxes the smooth muscles of the bronchi; eases breathing.

Cardiotonic Enhances heart function.

Carminative Induces the expulsion of gas.

Cathartic Rapidly brings about bowel eliminations.

Cholagogue Increases bile flow.

Choleretic *See* cholagogue.

Demulcent Soothing to irritated tissues. Used for sore throats and upset stomachs.

Deobstruent Clears obstructions from the body's ducts.

Depurant Helps to cleanse internal systems such as the intestinal tract, circulatory system, and urinary tract.

Depurgative Tends to bring about purification or cleansing.

Diaphoretic Stimulates perspiration; aids in eliminating wastes.

Disinfectant An agent that destroys or neutralizes the growth of disease-causing microorganisms.

Diuretic Increases amount of urine discharged.

Eliminative Encourages elimination of bodily wastes through the colon, kidneys, lymph, and skin.

Emetic Causes vomiting.

Emmenagogue Promotes menstruation.

Emollient Used to soothe the skin.

Expectorant Aids in the discharge of mucus and phlegm from the lungs and throat.

Febrifuge See antipyretic.

Galactagogue Stimulates lactation.

Hemostatic Stops bleeding.

Hepatic Beneficial to the liver.

Hypotensive Tends to lower the blood pressure.

Immunotonic Strengthens the immune system by increasing the production of white blood cells, hormones, and enzymes.

Laxative Brings about bowel movements.

Lythontryptic Urinary tract disinfectant.

Nephritic   Used to treat kidney problems.

Nervine   Used to calm nervous conditions.

Ophthalmic   Used to treat the eyes.

Oxytocic   Intensifies labor and speeds childbirth.

Parturient   *See* oxytocic.

Phytohormone   A hormone produced by a plant; plant hormones control such physiological functions as germination, growth, and metabolism.

Potentiator   An herb that increases the action of another herb.

Purgative   Brings about radical bowel evacuation.

Rubefacient   Substances that irritate the skin, producing redness.

Salivant   Stimulates secretion of saliva.

Secretagogue   Stimulates secretion of vital bodily fluids.

Sedative   Reduces anxiety, stress, or excitement.

Somnifacient   Sleep inducing.

Spasmolytic   Relieving or preventing spasms.

Stimulant   Temporarily arouses physiological activity.

Stomachic   Stimulates the production of digestive juices; relieves gastric disorders.

Styptic   Stops bleeding.

Sudorific   Induces or increases perspiration.

Sympathomimetic   Produces physiological effects that resemble those caused by the sympathetic nervous system (i.e., reduction of digestive secretions, contraction of blood vessels, increase in heart rate).

Tonic   Invigorates, refreshes, or restores the whole body.

Vasodilator   Expands blood vessels; promotes circulation.

Vermifuge   Expels worms from the intestines.

Vulnerary   A substance used to treat wounds.

The following list summarizes some common disorders that may be amenable to herbal interventions. The herbal substances in the table were selected because some data exists that may permit a reasonable standardization of the active compounds in a preparation or extract.

Common Conditions and the Herbs Used to Treat Them

Alzheimer's disease   St. John's wort, Ginko biloba

Asthma   Aniseed, celandine, licorice root, valerian

Blood pressure   Mistletoe, garlic, ginger

Boils	Chamomile, marjoram, marsh mallow, nasturtium, sanicle, compress of thyme
Bronchitis	Comfrey, camphor
Burns	Raw onions, potatoes, and aloe
Cholesterol (high)	Guggulipid, soybean extract (isoflavones)
Colds	Andrographis, chamomile inhalations, cinnamon, echinacea, ginger, marjoram infusions, peppermint, sunflower seed oil, thyme, yarrow
Constipation	Calamint, elder blossom, hyssop, peppermint
Depression	St. John's wort
Diarrhea	Infusion of blackberry root, cinnamon, peppermint, peppers
Dyspepsia	Caraway, fennel, peppermint
Fatigue	Agrimony, marjoram, peppermint, rose hips, yeast tablets
Fevers	Andrographis, tinctures of aconite, feverfew
Flatulence	Caraway, tincture of cardamom, charcoal biscuits, fennel, garlic, tumeric
Gout	Colchium, hyssop, juniper, capsicum
Headache	Chamomile, lavender (topically), mint, poppy
Heart disease	Andrographis, foxglove, motherwort
Insomnia	Aniseed, bergamot, hops, valerian
Immune disorders	Andrographis, echinacea, garlic
Menstrual problems	Lady's mantle tea, mistletoe, rose hips
Piles	Lesser celandine, plantain (pulped leaves applied locally)
Rheumatism	Boswellia, chamomile, hyssop, mugwort, onion (rubbed on joints), rosemary (externally)
Sore throat	Stinging nettle (gargled), honey
Sprains and bruises	Arnica (externally), bromelain
Stings and bites	Horseradish (externally), dock leaves (topically)
Stomach ulcers	Boswellia, garlic, licorice, peppermint
Toothache	Oil of cloves, elder, tansy

Urinary disorders	Bearberry, birch, chamomile, infusion of chickweed, cowberry, saw palmetto, *Pygeum africanum*, stinging nettles
Varicose veins	Fresh coltsfoot leaves in a poultice, valerian
Vomiting	Chamomile, peppermint, spearmint, rhubarb

A to Z Guide to Commonly Used Herbs

Alfalfa (*Medicago sativa*)

Alfalfa has been used to lower cholesterol, promote good circulation, treat diabetes and provide general stimulating effects as a tonic and a promoter of appetite. Alfalfa is quite nutritious, containing fiber, protein, unsaturated fatty acids, calcium, phosphorus, iron, other trace elements, organic acids, and vitamins K and C, together with chlorophyll pigment. Evidence for its benefit in the promotion of health is quite scant. Alfalfa should be taken in moderation because some evidence exists that it may cause blood abnormalities, such as a form of anemia and lupus. In fact, alfalfa should probably be avoided by those who have autoimmune diseases.

Aloe (*Aloe barbadenis*)

Aloe is used in the treatment of immune deficiency, diabetes mellitus, cancer, asthma, and AIDS. It has a long history of use as a topical agent for a variety of dermatological problems. More recently, aloe products have become the focus of intensive multi-level marketing activity; aloe products are ubiquitous in health food stores and grocery stores. Aloe is very beneficial in the topical treatment of abrasions, burns (especially sunburn), and dry skin. While the evidence for aloe as a therapeutic agent in a variety of skin disorders is quite convincing, the evidence for the oral use of aloe in several disease states remains very questionable.

Contemporary research has focused on the presence of chemicals called acemannans as important active compounds in aloe preparations. There is some evidence that they may exert a beneficial effect on immune function. Perhaps the most convincing evidence of benefit of the oral administration of aloe vera comes from limited and anecdotal studies on the value of acemannans, which have been used in doses of approximately 1 gm per day to enhance body immunity. In order to obtain this much acemannan from many commercial types of aloe, an individual may have to consume very large quantities of aloe extracts or juice.

There is limited evidence that aloe has been useful as a complementary therapy in the treatment of AIDS, with some reports of synergistic effects with AZT. The postulated antiviral effects of acemannans require further clarification. Unfortunately, claims that aloe is a body cleanser, antiseptic, fever-reducing agent, nutrient, or anti-inflammatory agent are not supported conclusively by controlled studies or clinical information, but anecdotal benefit is apparent.

There are multiple sources of aloe, but the two main sources are aloe vera gels, prepared from the leaf of the plant, and aloe juice, or latex, which may be derived from dried plants or plants treated by a variety of chemical or mechanical processes. It has been observed that many aloe preparations may lose their "activity" if stored. Several dietary supplement manufacturers claim that their type of aloe extract contains active ingredients without showing much evidence of health benefits.

You should also be aware that the word *aloe* can be applied to commercial products that contain minimal amounts of putative, active constituents. Many aloe products are reconstituted from extracts or concentrates of variably prepared derivatives of aloe.

Angelica (*Angelica archangelica*)

Angelica, which is variably produced from the root, stem, leaves, or fruits of angelica plants, has been used in folklore medicine in the belief that it prevented gas and encouraged the passage of perspiration and urine. There is little evidence to support that angelica has these functions. Angelica has been used to induce abortion, and if used in large doses in these circumstances, it is very dangerous. Extracts of angelica contain compounds that may make the skin more susceptible to damage by sunlight. This susceptibility is called photosensitivity. Angelica and related herbs from this genus of plants should not be used for self-medication.

Apricot Pits (Laetrile)

Laetrile — commonly compounded of extracts from apricot kernels — was a very popular alternative cancer cure in the 1960s and 1970s. Several research studies subsequently brought into question the efficacy of laetrile and related compounds in cancer therapy.

The Food and Drug Administration took sanctions against the sale of laetrile in 1971, but it was not until the 1980's that multicenter clinical trials were performed with laetrile by the National Cancer Institute. These studies concluded that laetrile may be ineffective in cancer therapy. Today, laetrile is not commonly used in the United States, but it is still used and touted as a cancer cure by clinics in adjacent countries. Although the alternative medicine community has taken issue with the conclusions of the clinical trials performed by the National Cancer Institute, there is, at present, no solid evidence that amygdalin (the compound in apricot pits) or "laetrile" in any form has measurable benefit in the treatment of cancer.

Barberry (*Berberis vulgaris*)

Barberry is a Native American remedy that is said to be a general tonic. It contains alkaloids of uncertain pharmacological effects and probably has little place in contemporary herbal therapy.

Bayberry (*Myrica cerifera*)

Bayberry root and bark contain compounds that may have steroidlike effects, but some concern exists about bayberry's ability to cause cancer in experimental animals. Bayberry may have some health benefits, but its safety is questionable.

Betony (*Stachys officinalis*)

Betony was formerly used as a health panacea, but its only real value is as an astringent. Its astringency comes from the chemical tannin, which is used in the tanning of hides. Betony as a mouthwash has some use for gingivitis, and the herb has been reported to be effective in the management of some types of diarrhea.

Bilberry (*Vaccinium myrtillus*)

Much interest exists in the use of bilberry extracts that contain chemicals (anthocyanosides or flavonoids) which are known to be antioxidants. Several studies have shown that anthocyanosides in bilberries can improve visual acuity at night and enhance the eye's ability to adapt to the dark. The herb's active components work on retinal cells, and favorable results of the administration of bilberry extracts have been reported in a variety of ocular disorders, including diabetic retinopathy, macular degeneration, and several causes of night blindness. British Royal Air Force pilots who used bilberry reported improvement in their nocturnal eyesight during bombing raids on Germany in World War II.

Bilberry is a component of several dietary supplements that are sold to promote ocular health. Standardized bilberry extracts have much to offer in ocular health. They remain under-investigated and under-applied in clinical practice.

Black and Blue Cohosh (*Cimicifuga racemosa* and *Caulophyllum thalictroides*)

Black and blue cohosh have similar names, but their effects on the body are like "chalk and cheese." Currently, black cohosh is being proposed as an herbal product for the relief of menopausal symptoms and premenstrual syndrome. There is evidence in animals that black cohosh may contain compounds that bind to estrogen receptors, but the evidence for estrogenic effects in humans remains debatable. Despite the few accounts of the safety of black cohosh, this herb is being used increasingly as a component of herbal supplements to promote a healthy menopause. The evidence to support the use of black cohosh as a menopausal supplement is miniscule in comparison to the well-documented evidence for the use of phytoestrogens, such as soy isoflavones, in the promotion of menopausal health.

Blue cohosh contains a variety of alkaloids and glycosides of poorly defined pharmaceutical effect, raising questions about the herb's safety. Descriptions of the use of cohosh in herbal medicine indicate an almost panacea benefit, but evidence for this is lacking.

Borage (*Borago officinalis*)

Borage is a classic astringent containing tannins. It has a reputation for relieving symptoms of depression. In addition, much interest has focused on borage oil as a source of health-giving unsaturated fatty acids (omega 6, essential fatty acids). Some borage oil contains certain alkaloids that may be carcinogenic or damage the liver. Only borage oil free of toxins should be used, and the chronic consumption of certain types of borage oil may not be healthy.

Boswellia (*Boswellia serrata*)

Boswellia is extracted from gum resins derived from the tree *Boswellia serrata*. The extract belongs to a class of compounds called guggals, which have been described in ancient Ayurvedic medicine as possessing potent, antirheumatic properties. The active ingredients of boswellia extract are beta-boswellic acid and other acids.

Many studies have confirmed the benefit of standardized boswellia extract in the treatment of osteoarthritis and rheumatoid arthritis. Boswellic acids can protect against artificially induced arthritis in animals; the herb's anti-inflammatory actions have been well documented in soft tissue inflammation. Detailed laboratory experiments have shown that extracts of boswellia serrata resin protect the main constituents of bone and cartilage (chondroitins) by reducing the activity of several enzymes that degrade important structural components of cartilage (glycosaminoglycans).

Some scientists have referred to boswellia as a nonsteroidal anti-inflammatory agent; this is not to be confused with standard nonsteroidal anti-inflammatory drugs (NSAIDs), such as ibuprofen and naproxen, which often cause stomach upset and may produce stomach or duodenal ulcers. It is notable that boswellia exhibits antiulcerogenic activity, in contrast to the ulcerogenic potential of NSAIDs.

Dietary supplements containing standardized extracts of boswellia have been reported repeatedly to reduce joint swelling and morning stiffness, increase joint mobility, and produce an overall improvement in quality of life. These effects have been seen in patients with a variety of rheumatological disorders such as: osteoarthritis, gouty arthritis, rheumatoid disease, nonspecific rheumatism, fibrositis, myositis, cervical spondylolysis, and backache due to vertebral disorders. Boswellia is finding an increasing role as a dietary supplement or a topical preparation in the treatment of arthritis in humans, dogs with hip dysplasia, and lame horses. The importance of the standardization of boswellia products for their content of boswellic acids and pentacyclic triterpene acids should not be underestimated.

Bromelain

Bromelain is a mixture of certain protein-digesting enzymes (proteolytic) that are found in the stems of pineapples. Recent collaborative studies by Dr. Holt and researchers at the University of Costa Rica show that most bromelain is contained in the stem of the pineapple nearest to the fruit. Concentrations of bromelain are also found in the woody core of pineapples.

There are more than one hundred scientific studies supporting the use of bromelain as potential therapy for arthritis, sports injuries, and soft tissue trauma. Bromelain has anti-inflammatory effects, including some demonstrated ability to block the production of compounds that mediate inflammation. Bromelain is sometimes a component of dietary supplements used to promote joint health, and the supporting evidence for this application is quite plausible.

Bran

Bran is a form of dietary fiber that has many potential health-giving properties. Dietary fiber resists digestion by the human gastrointestinal tract. Well-conducted epidemiologic, clinical, and experimental studies imply that bran supplementation can assist in the treatment or prevention of several diseases, including coronary heart disease, varicose veins, diverticular disease, and colon cancer. Bran has been used as a way of promoting a feeling of fullness in the treatment of obesity, and good evidence exists that it can lower blood cholesterol. Supplementation of the diet with approximately 20 gm of bran per day is effective treatment for irritable bowel syndrome.

Bran may interfere with the absorption of calcium and other essential minerals, but this occurrence is rarely of clinical significance. When bran is incorporated into an average diet, an individual often experiences abdominal bloating and excessive gas for a time. Many people stop using bran supplementation because of this. Furthermore, eating bran is sometimes like "chewing cardboard." Attempts to provide bran in more palatable formats have met with variable success.

No one should question the health benefits of bran, but many people reject it as a dietary supplement because it is difficult to take. The authors believe that one of the best ways to take bran is in a compressed tablet form. Be advised that you must consume adequate quantities of fluid when using bran supplements. Many of the beneficial effects of bran are related to its ability to hold water while it resides in the intestines.

Butcher's-broom (*Ruscus aculeatus*)

Butcher's-broom defies clear definition because different plants have been used to produce several products that bear the name butcher's-broom. Extracts of stems of certain types of butcher's-broom contain compounds that affect blood vessels which appear to work on receptors in the adrenergic nervous system. These agents are believed by some to be beneficial in assisting in the restoration of vessel tone, especially in the lower limbs.

Butcher's-broom has been used to promote beneficial effects on the circulation. The overall effect of this herb is to cause constriction of blood vessels. Self-medication with butcher's-broom cannot be recommended because vasoconstriction can have serious consequences.

Caffeine-Containing Products

Caffeine is ubiquitous in the American diet and it is addictive. Herbals or beverages containing caffeine are best taken in moderation. The recent practice of combining ephedrine and caffeine in diet pills is dangerous and ill advised.

There is no argument that caffeine has potent pharmacological effects, especially stimulatory effects. Individuals with healthy hearts as well as those with heart disease may suffer irregular heartbeat as a consequence of consuming caffeine. Many people forget that caffeine can cause nervousness, anxiety, insomnia, excess stomach acidity, high blood glucose, and high cholesterol levels. Furthermore, the lay public is not universally aware that caffeine can cause deformities in the fetuses of experimental animals. Pregnant women should severely limit their caffeine intake.

Calendula (*Calendula officinalis*)

Calendula is an ancient remedy that has unequivocal benefit when applied topically to assist in wound healing and the management of dry and chapped skin. Amazingly, relatively little research has been done with topical calendula, despite the continuous reporting of its beneficial effects.

Capsicum (*Capsicum frutescens*) or Cayenne

Capsicum is found in several different types of pepper, and it is used both in topical and oral forms. The active ingredient of capsicum is capsaicin, which may have stimulatory effects on gastrointestinal function, anti-clotting effects, and cholesterol-lowering ability. It is believed that capsaicin depletes a particular substance (substance P) that facilitates the transmission of pain through peripheral nerves. Capsaicin is used to control the pain of skin eruptions, such as cold sores or herpes.

Capsicum can be applied topically as a counter-irritant. When taken orally, it has variable effects. It may even protect against peptic ulceration, although spices in the diet may exacerbate symptoms of peptic ulcer disease. Capsicum should be used under medical supervision because dosage is uncertain. People with a hiatus hernia or gastrointestinal problems should avoid cayenne (capsicum).

Chaparral (*Larrea tridentata*)

Chaparral is mentioned because of its historical interest. This plant grows wild in many Southwestern states in the United States and is an old Native American remedy for just about every disease. Chaparral contains a substance (nordihydroguaiaretic acid) that some believe can cure cancer. Because this component of chaparral is very toxic, certain preparations of this herb should not be consumed by humans.

Comfrey (*Symphytum officinale*)

Comfrey has been used mainly in topical applications as a poultice for wound healing. It may be toxic when taken internally, and preparations of comfrey may be contaminated with compounds derived from deadly night-shade. The most significant problem associated with comfrey ingestion is the possibility of liver toxicity believed to be related to its content of certain alkaloids. The FDA considers comfrey to be unsafe for internal use.

Cranberry (*Vaccinium macrocarpon*)

Extracts of cranberry, whole cranberries, and cranberry juice are widely promoted for their benefit in the management of urinary tract infection and kidney stones. The beneficial effect of cranberry in urinary tract infection has been documented.

Certain components of cranberries have antibacterial properties. These components seem to prevent bacteria from sticking to cells that line the urinary tract. Because cranberry juice is acidic (it contains hippuric acid), large amounts can cause acidification of the urine. This does not appear to be the main mechanism for the beneficial effect of cranberry in urinary tract infection.

Curcumin

Curcumin is is the yellow pigment of *Curcuma longa,* or turmeric, a spice used in the preparation of Indian curry. Curcumin is known to be an effective anti-inflammatory substance. Animal experiments show that turmeric has anticancer effects, and several human studies are underway to assess the anticancer potential of turmeric.

Dandelion (*Taraxacum officinale*)

Dandelion has enjoyed widespread use in the treatment of a host of conditions. Its use in folklore medicine is not supported by much scientific research. Dandelion appears safe but innocuous.

Devil's Claw (*Harpagophytum procumbens*)

Devil's claw may be useful as an appetite stimulant and carminative (flatulence-reducing substance). It is used widely in several European countries and is touted as a cure for many chronic degenerative diseases. Some practitioners of herbal medicine believe that this herb has antirheumatic properties, but supporting data is limited.

Dong Quai (*Angelica senensis*)

Dong quai is the classic female herbal supplement. It must not be used in pregnancy, but it has many reports of successful use in the treatment of painful menstruation, premenstrual syndrome, and menopausal symptoms. It is believed that dong quai can have a modulating effect on the activity of estrogen. This herb may contain compounds that can make people sensitive to light, and some residual concerns about safety exist. Dong quai is used widely in Asia and is a principal component of several traditional Chinese and Ayurvedic medicines.

Echinacea (*Echinacea angustifolia*)

The North American Indians have used echinacea for centuries. Today, echinacea is a staple dietary supplement that is widely used in North America and Europe as an alternative treatment for cancer, as a treatment of yeast infections, and for enhancement of immunity and wound healing. Most of the research on echinacea has been performed in Europe, even though the plants from which this herb is derived are native to North America. There is sound scientific agreement that the herb contains compounds which stimulate the immune system in a variety of ways. (See pages 90–93 for additional information and Appendix A for more technical information.) Data supporting the use of echinacea to enhance the body's defenses is so strong that the German government has recommended the herb be used as supportive therapy for a variety of recurrent infections. Echinacea is here to stay with evidence of benefit, even if some of the claims are overstated.

The reader should remember that all types of echinacea are not "born equal" in terms of their biological effects (see page 91).

Ephedra (*Ephedra sinica*)

Ephedra is an ancient Chinese remedy that is often used in the treatment of respiratory illness and allergy. The active constituents of ephedra — known as *ma huang* in China — are ephedrine and related compounds. These compounds form the basis of commonly used, modern over-the-counter cough and cold remedies (e.g., pseudoephedrine). In high doses, ephedra can excite the mind and stimulate the central nervous system. It can raise blood pressure, increase heart rate, and cause insomnia and mental agitation. *Ma huang* should not be used in conjunction with caffeine. It is best to limit your daily intake of this herb to 40 milligrams or less. Ephedra should not be used by individuals with significant heart disease or high blood pressure.

Young people have very foolishly used the herb to enhance athletic performance or as an illicit drug. Controls now exist on the use of *ma huang* in some states.

There would appear to be little advantage for health in the components of *ma huang* other than its content of ephedrine. Since ephedrine is freely available in a standardized format, a good argument exists to ban the use of *ma huang* completely. Unfortunately, this ban will not prevent individuals from abusing over-the-counter sources of ephedrine in their quest for a short-lived but dangerous high.

Evening Primrose (*Oenothera biennis*)

Evening primrose oil has built some of the largest dietary supplement companies in the industry. A great deal of literature supports the potential benefit of the fatty acid components of this oil in the treatment of premenstrual tension, menopausal symptoms, diabetic kidney disease, and even attention deficit disorder (ADD) in children. Each manufacturer of evening primrose oil claims its product is better than the others. The evidence for superiority is variable.

Evening primrose oil's health-giving constituent appears to be a precursor of a hormonelike substance that mediates such physiological functions as metabolism, smooth muscle activity, and nerve transmission. While some nutritionists rave about evening primrose oil and its benefit, other oils of plant origin (e.g., soybean, safflower, pumpkin seed, and black currant) also have potential benefits in terms of their essential fatty acids.

In Western society, most people's diets are deficient in omega-3 fatty acids, which are found predominantly in fish oil. Although some plants contain precursors of these fatty acids, there is doubt that they can be effectively utilized by the body to produce the previously mentioned hormonelike substances (prostaglandins). Evening primrose oil may have been overrated as a health-giving dietary supplement. It can be speculated that equal research into fish oil would reveal more evidence of health benefit than that obtained from evening primrose oil.

Fennel (*Foeniculum vulgare*)

Fennel is a classic carminative (flatulence reducer). It is used with peppermint oil in a delayed release formula to treat irritable bowel syndrome and lower digestive upset. Safe in small doses, fennel relaxes smooth muscle in the gut. (See Appendix A for technical details.) Sugar-coated fennel seeds are commonly taken after a meal in India to stop halitosis and promote digestion.

Feverfew (*Tanacetum parthenium*)

Feverfew is used by some herbalists to treat nonspecific headache, abdominal pain, and fevers. As the name suggests, much anecdotal evidence supports feverfew's ability to reduce fevers. Several double-blind, controlled studies indicate that feverfew may be a useful treatment for headaches of diverse causes.

One of the most interesting applications of this herb is in both the prevention and treatment of migraine headaches. Its precise mechanism of action in this circumstance remains to be defined, but some evidence suggests that this herb may assist in normalizing blood vessel tone by modulating the release of vasoactive compounds in the body. The active ingredient of feverfew is believed to be parthenolide.

Fo-Ti (*Polygonum multiflorum*)

Fo-ti, known as *ho shou wu* in China, may be useful in bringing about bowel evacuation, though its long list of potential beneficial health effects has defied plausible documentation, despite its longtime use in traditional Chinese medical practice. There is some evidence that fractions of fo-ti may be beneficial in treating circulatory disorders such as inadequate blood flow in veins. The herb has been used for nocturnal cramps in the lower limbs and in the management of heavy legs syndrome, a condition of doubtful cause.

Garlic (*Allium sativum*)

Garlic is a very popular dietary supplement; it is, in fact, the number-one selling dietary supplement in the United States. Garlic has unequivocally beneficial effects on cardiovascular health.

Garlic seems to be very versatile in its ability to promote health, and a voluminous amount of literature exists to support its use.

Ginger (*Zingiber officinale*)

Ginger is a carminative (flatulence reducer), and it has value in the treatment of motion sickness. It can be taken in several forms but seems to exert most benefit when taken as a capsule containing high quality ginger powder. The active constituents of ginger still remain a mystery, although herbalists talk about gingerosides as though they are well-defined and well-studied compounds.

Ginko (*Ginko biloba*)

Ginko biloba has taken the dietary supplement market by storm. Ginko has a long history of use in traditional Chinese medicine. It is most commonly used in Western society for its potential benefits in the treatment of artery blockages caused by tumorlike growths, the treatment of asthma, and the management of Alzheimer's disease and other types of dementia. Ginko is used very commonly by German physicians, and many scientific studies provide good evidence that ginko can exert beneficial effects on blood circulation. Of most significance are studies that show improved cerebral circulation in the elderly. Ginko is rapidly finding a role in modern conventional and alternative medical practice.

Ginseng, American (*Panax quinquefolium*) and
Ginseng, Asian (*Panax ginseng*)

Ginseng is regarded as a panacea of health. It is regarded as a classic adaptogen and a general tonic. It is also believed that the herb can enhance the body's ability to ward off disease. Unfortunately, finding standardized or authentic ginseng is very difficult.

The story of ginseng and health typifies one of the major problems in the dietary supplement industry. Several studies performed with one type of ginseng or an extract may show unequivocal benefit. These studies are then quoted as support for the sale of other types of ginseng. Favorable reports about one type of herb, grown in a specific location and manufactured in a certain way, do not constitute evidence supporting the benefit of all ginseng products as dietary supplements.

Ginseng appears to be generally safe, although arguments prevail as to whether adverse effects occur following the use of "average" amounts of ginseng as a dietary supplement. Manufacturers of various ginseng products must focus their studies on demonstrating that their brand or preparation has biological activity and reasonable consistency. Unfortunately, quality is not the guideword for a significant sector of the dietary supplement industry.

Goldenseal (*Hydrastis canadensis*)

Goldenseal is a Native American remedy that has been used to treat infections, cancer, and liver disease. Goldenseal is combined with echinacea in some dietary supplements. It has been proposed that goldenseal has beneficial effects on mucous membranes lining several body cavities. This herb may exert some benefit on infectious diarrhea, but well controlled studies are lacking.

Some individuals think they can cheat drug-screening blood or urine tests by taking goldenseal. They are mistaken.

Gotu Kola (*Centella asiatica*)

Large doses of gotu kola may cause an individual to fall asleep. Claims that the herb promotes longevity have no scientific support.

Guggulipid

Guggulipid is an extract of a tree resin that has been widely used in Ayurvedic medicine to promote cardiovascular health and treat rheumatic disorders. A significant number of controlled clinical studies show that guggulipid can lower blood cholesterol. The active constituents of guggulipid are called guggulsterones. This Ayurvedic resin's effect on lowering blood cholesterol can be enhanced by adding vitamin C.

Dietary supplements of guggulipid should only be used if they are standardized. Guggulipid appears quite safe.

Hawthorne

Hawthorne is emerging as a herbal preparation for the treatment of cardiac and circulatory system disorders. Some studies imply that it may be useful in the treatment of angina and it may be safe at recommended doses if standardized extracts are used. Hawthorne may lower blood pressure by inhibiting certain enzymes, in a fashion similar to commonly used antihypertensive medications. Self-medication with hawthorne in the presence of significant cardiac disease is not recommended.

Licorice (*Glycyrrhiza glabra*)

Licorice has been used to treat peptic ulcer, menopausal symptoms, liver disease, inflammatory conditions, and even AIDS. Many studies of licorice imply that the herb can, in certain formats, heal peptic ulcer disease. There is little evidence for the benefit of licorice in the treatment of disease other than peptic ulcer. Unfortunately, licorice contains steroidlike molecules that cause fluid retention, swelling (edema), and high blood pressure. Do not use it if you have high blood pressure.

Licorice is commonly found in candy, but large amounts of candy containing licorice may result in toxicity, especially in the elderly. A preparation called deglycyrrhizinated licorice was marketed as an approved ulcer healing remedy, but its use has been superseded by more effective and safer treatments.

Milk Thistle (*Cardus marianus*)

Milk thistle is used by herbalists for liver disease, and some evidence exists that it may protect the liver against a variety of toxins. The active ingredient of milk thistle is silymaron, a flavonoid that has shown some benefit in limited human clinical trials in patients with hepatitis and cirrhosis. Milk thistle appears safe.

Mistletoe (*Viscum album*)

Mistletoe is good for eliciting kisses, but it is quite toxic when taken orally. The toxicity of mistletoe varies by species or hybrid. It has untoward effects on the cardiovascular system and should be avoided.

Myrrh (*Commiphora myrrha*)

Myrrh finds its greatest use in perfumes and incense. It may be useful as an expensive astringent when applied topically. It has little use in health care.

Nettles (*Urtica urens*)

In general, nettles are very interesting plants. Stinging nettle is a significant and apparently effective component of natural remedies for prostate enlargement. Several clinical trials support the use of stinging nettles in the management of prostatic disease. Based on this evidence, several European countries have recommended that stinging nettle be used as a standard therapeutic agent for prostate disorders.

Papaya (*Carica papaya*)

Papaya is a delicious fruit that contains a mixed bag of enzymes which digest protein. The mixture of enzymes is referred to as papain, which, because of its ability to digest protein, is used in meat tenderizers. Papain deserves more study as an enzyme supplement to promote digestive health. Papaya has been promoted in encapsulated dietary supplements as a digestive aid. There are few studies in humans showing the effects of papaya, but clinical assessments show symptomatic benefit in individuals with a variety of digestive disturbances. Since the proposed benefit of papaya supplements is related to the enzymes it contains, only products that have consistent enzymatic activity should be used.

Topical application of papaya is said to assist in removing skin blemishes, unclogging pores, and generally cleansing the skin.

Parsley (*Petroselinum sativum*)

Parsley is an antiflatulent that also induces the expulsion of gas. It may have some diuretic (increasing the flow of urine) effects. Some components of the oils contained within parsley are toxic and should not be used in pregnancy because they may induce abortion. Parsley has been incorporated into some supplements that may freshen the breath. Extracts of parsley are safe in small doses but possibly dangerous in large ones.

Pollen

Pollen has been used to treat almost every chronic disease known to man. Since 1920, it has been highly regarded as a cure for allergies. There is no question that pollen is a treasure chest of nutrients and bioactive compounds, and pollen of various types is available in dietary supplement formats. Many types of pollen can cause allergic reactions, some of which can be very serious. Unfortunately, pollen defies standardization because the "active constituents" of pollen, if they exist, are not well defined. Overall, there is not a great deal of good scientific evidence that pollen has specific health benefits. Many herbalists still espouse its benefits.

Propolis

Propolis is a substance that bees collect from the buds of certain trees and use as "cement" in their hives. It has demonstrable antibacterial and antifungal effects, which tend to be weaker than antibiotics. Propolis is often marketed in combination with pollen in the form of tablets or capsules. Evidence for a benefit for either of these substances in well controlled clinical studies is not readily available.

Pycnogenol and Related Compounds

Called OPC by medical researchers, pycnogenol and related mixtures of flavonoids are a mixture of antioxidant molecules. These botanical "vitamin C helpers" have become very popular as dietary supplements because of their potent and versatile biological effects, including antioxidant effects.

Used experimentally in antiaging medicines, these agents have been applied to the treatment of every chronic degenerative disease known to man. Their value as isolated therapeutic agents is doubted by practitioners of conventional medicine. While their application to many disease states has aroused healthy skepticism, good scientific agreement exists that they play a major role in the maintenance of collagen and other supporting tissues in the body. The authors believe that they may have some role to play in the maintenance of general health, but more controlled clinical studies are required.

Royal Jelly

Secreted by worker bees, royal jelly is the food of queen bees. Perhaps because queen bees live about twenty times longer than other bees in the hive, royal jelly is believed to have antiaging properties. Royal jelly has been proposed as an aphrodisiac and general tonic. It probably does not restore hair, but it has been known to cause allergic reactions. Royal jelly undoubtedly contains many interesting nutrients and compounds, which still require definition.

St. John's Wort (*Hypericum perforatum*)

At the time of this writing, St. John's wort is one of the most popular selling dietary supplements. Given the existing evidence of its benefit in depressive illness, the herb is of great interest. It is believed to have antidepressant effects and is proposed as an alternative to antidepressant medication. Recently, Duke University in North Carolina received a large government grant to study the chemistry and health application of St. John's wort.

Unfortunately, many types of St. John's wort are available for sale, but the content of active agents is not standardized. (See Appendix A for technical information on active agents.) The herb appears quite safe at recommended doses, but the long-term safety of St. John's wort is not known. Cases of hypersensitivity and photosensitivity have been reported with its use.

Saw Palmetto (*Serenoa serrulata*)

Considerable evidence has accrued that extracts of saw palmetto may be useful in the treatment of prostatic disease. This herb is used in several countries as a prescription medication for the treatment of benign enlargement of the prostate. Although several regulatory agencies in the United States have accepted evidence of saw palmetto's benefit in the treatment of prostatic disease, the Food and Drug Administration remains unwilling to accept its efficacy. There is some concern that only certain fractions of saw palmetto are active. Practitioners of complementary medicine remain convinced that several herbal extracts of saw palmetto or preparations of the whole herb are effective in the management of prostatic enlargement.

Senna (*Cassia senna*)

Senna enjoys widespread but sometimes reckless use as a purgative, a substance that brings about radical bowel evacuation. Although the herb can be used safely on an infrequent basis, its chronic use can irreparably damage the colon by producing a disorder called cathartic colon.

Senna has appealed to some misguided people who think that their bowel must be emptied at least once or more in a twenty-four-hour period. Such individuals fail to recognize that the range of normal bowel habit is from three bowel actions per day to one bowel action every three days. To force the colon to empty unnecessarily is not good practice. Irregularities of bowel habit in the absence of disease are best managed by lifestyle changes, such as increased exercise and more consumption of fluids, fruits, and vegetables. Supplementation of the diet with fiber such as bran is also a good idea.

Skullcap (*Scutellaria lateriflora*)

Skullcap is used for a variety of central nervous system diseases, but it is best known for its tranquilizing effects. There is some concern that extracts of skullcap may have toxic effects, especially liver damage. Unfortunately, there seems to be little general agreement about the best source of skullcap and even less agreement about its active constituents.

Soy Isoflavones

Isoflavones found in soybeans are an example of estrogens derived from plants. The principal soy isoflavones (genistein and daidzein) bear a structural resemblance to the female hormone estrogen and can modulate its effects. Potent biological agents, soy isoflavones also have demonstrable anticancer effects and antioxidant effects in animals and humans. (For more information on the anticancer benefits of soy, see Chapter 7.)

Spirulina (Blue-Green Algae)

Spirulina, a good source of a variety of nutrients, has been used, with alleged success, as a weight loss aid. It seems to have a high concentration of the amino acid phenylalanine, which has been touted inappropriately as an appetite suppressant. Spirulina may be good food, but evidence that it has versatile health benefits is lacking.

Tea Tree Oil (*Melaleuca alternifolia*)

Incorporated into a variety of creams and lotions, tea tree oil has been used topically for wound healing and as an antiseptic. It appears to have widespread antimicrobial activity. Tea tree oil, however, may trigger allergic skin rashes. Overall, it is effective when applied topically to minor skin disorders, but other more potent and more specific remedies are available.

Valerian (*Valeriana officinalis*)

Valerian root is an herbal sedative that has been used as a sleep aid. This herb is used quite commonly in Germany as a treatment for insomnia, and it is regarded as a tranquilizer. It appears that valerian is quite safe and it has much to offer as a first-line option before an individual takes a tranquilizer of synthetic origin.

Yohimbe (*Pausinystalia yohimbe*)

Yohimbe is regarded as an aphrodisiac and is being used increasingly by elderly males who wish to retain their sexual vitality. The herb, made from the bark of trees that grow in central Africa, does have stimulant and potential hallucinogenic activity. The active agent may have an effect on the transmission of certain nerve impulses, but it may cause excitation and induce agitation or anxiety. Some have expressed concern about yohimbe's potential to cause serious adverse effects. Still, this herb is sold widely in "raunchy" magazines, some herbal stores, and sex shops. Yohimbe should not be rejected as lacking in any potential use because there are few effective agents to treat impotence of unknown origin. Further study is required to assess its efficacy and safety.

Marine Nutriceuticals

The following dietary supplements of marine origin are included here because they have been combined with herbs or botanicals in some commonly used products.

Kelp

Kelp is a vague term that describes many types of seaweed. Many studies allege the benefit of kelp in a variety of disease states. A review of such studies by regulatory authorities in Germany and the United States has not resulted in any recommendation for a specific health benefit of kelp.

New Zealand Green-Lipped Mussel

The New Zealand green-lipped mussel has been used alone or in combination with herbal products to treat arthritis. Several studies have examined the role of extracts of this mussel in arthritis treatment, but data are conflicting.

Shark Cartilage

Shark cartilage has become the most popular alternative cancer therapy since the use of laetrile. Considerable debate exists over the potential benefit of shark cartilage in the treatment of cancer. Evidence to date does not support the notion that shark cartilage is a cancer cure, even though it may have some yet-to-be-defined benefit in some patients with cancer. It appears that certain types of pure shark cartilage may exert an antiangiogenic effect and interfere with unwanted blood vessel growth, which is a major cause of several common, chronic diseases.

Some evidence has emerged that shark cartilage may be useful in the promotion of bone and joint health when administered orally as a dietary supplement. Evidence also exists that shark cartilage has much to offer as a topical agent in the management of burns or wounds that are difficult to heal.

Conclusion

The safety of many herbs remains in question, and dosing is arbitrary. The authors stress that self-medication with herbs is not advisable. The conclusions reached in the above summaries represent the authors' assessment of medical and folklore literature. Limitations of interpretation exist because complete research on even a few commonly used herbs is very difficult. Much information on the health benefits of herbs is anecdotal, and where possible this has been pointed out.

Dr. Holt has drawn upon his personal observations of the use of certain herbal treatments and has analyzed information found in many Western textbooks on herbs. One of the most balanced accounts of the use of botanical and herbal products as remedies is to be found in the book *The Honest Herbal* by Professor Varro E. Tyler, Ph.D. (Pharmaceutical Products Press, Haworth Press, Inc., New York). Now in its third edition, the book provides a great deal of information on studies to assess the benefit, or lack thereof, of many commonly used herbal products. The title of Professor Tyler's book — *The Honest Herbal* — may be unfortunate, because it may imply that other books on herbal remedies are dishonest. Although herbal medicine sometimes may be practiced by scoundrels and scalliwags, it is an art, and through history much of its application has involved empiric activity.

Those wishing to search the literature for additional information on the potential biological action of a specific herbal product can consult the annotated bibliography at the end of this book.

11

Preparing Herbal Remedies

Today's "green revolution" has led many people back to herbs, but Americans — at least since that fateful day in Boston — are traditionally coffee drinkers and probably don't know a lot about tea leaves or other herbs. Because the green revolution is still new, Americans may not have access to information about turning crude botanicals into viable therapies.

It is important to realize that some herbs in small doses are quite safe, but when the same herbs are given in larger doses, they may be quite toxic. Although herbs are of natural origin, they are not necessarily safe. Practitioners of herbal medicine have been criticized for generally recommending that all herbal products used in treatment are safe, though many practitioners of herbal medicine behave responsibly in their attitude toward the safety issues that surround the use of herbal agents.

It has been argued by many proponents of herbal therapy that there are relatively few examples of fatalities or serious side effects from the use of herbal products. For example, data from the American Association of Poison Control Centers reveals that between 1983 and 1990 there were more than two thousand deaths associated with prescription or over-the-counter drugs, as compared to only one death associated with vitamin supplements. The data may, however, be misleading and may paint too optimistic a picture of the safety of nutrient supplements.

In some circumstances in Western society, data on the adverse effects are derived from a voluntary reporting system among health care professionals. The relatively scarce records of adverse effects or deaths from the use of herbs is no guarantee that such occurrences are rare. The increasing and widespread use of herbal remedies may necessitate the establishment of formal postmarketing surveillance like that currently used to monitor the safety of ethical pharmaceuticals. Unfortunately, the dietary supplement industry is not obligated to collect prospective data about the safety of its products.

In general terms, herbal medicine is to be avoided in pregnancy and childhood because there is still relatively little information about its safety in these circumstances. The abortifacient (abortion inducing) or terato-genic (growth deforming) or carcinogenic (cancer causing) potential of some herbals and botanicals should not be underestimated.

The explosion in demand for herbal products has created a window of opportunity for some manufacturers to purvey herbs with hyped claims of health benefits. Many of these agents are now available as dietary supple-ments, and variable claims of health benefits are associated with them.

In most countries, dietary supplements cannot be used to diagnose, prevent, or treat any disease. Legislation passed in the United States in 1994 (the Dietary Supplement and Health Education Act), permits the sale of these products with "body-structure-function claims." Manufac-turers can tell consumers that a product affects a particular bodily structure or action, but they may not say that the herb treats, cures, or ameliorates any disease or condition. In other words, dealers and manufacturers can say, for example, that an herb dilates blood vessels, but they cannot say that it lowers blood pressure. These claims are meant to be part of an honest labeling process. (The importance of the regulation of health claims pertaining to dietary supplements is summarized in Appendix B.)

Unfortunately, due to a lack of standardization in the dietary supplement industry, there is no guarantee that some herbal products have biological activity. Furthermore, there are doubts regarding the consistency of herbal products from batch to batch, even when they are sold under the same brand name.

A number of dietary supplement manufacturers have attempted to standardize products. These companies include Nature's Way (Murdoch, Madaus, Schwabe, Inc.) of Springville, Utah, and BioTherapies, Inc., of Fairfield, New Jersey. (A listing of these and other companies begins on page 196).

Before you can begin preparing your own herbal remedies, there is much more you need to know. The preparation of herbal remedies is only recommended for the enthusiast, with knowledge, disposable time, and commitment.

Preparing Therapies From Botanicals

Natural substances that have undergone no processing beyond collecting and drying are referred to as crude botanicals. These include plants, herbs, and saps that have not been shredded, ground, chipped, distilled, evaporated, or mixed with other substances. On the opposite end of the spectrum are products that are considered advanced. These have undergone physical or mechanical processing to enhance their value or improve their quality.

Crude botanicals are rarely used as therapeutic agents. There are, however, many ways to turn these materials into herbal remedies. Most of these have been developed through trial and error during centuries of use. In the manufacture of pharmaceuticals, active components of botanicals are normally isolated, identified, and then synthesized. Herbalists also separate active components from the botanical. These components are then known as derivatives or extracts. Extraction removes substances that can be dissolved in a liquid known as a solvent. After extraction, an undissolved portion of the crude botanical remains. Known as the marc, this residue is discarded.

In vast experience using herbs, herbalists have learned that some botanicals have more therapeutic value when used as decoctions, while some medicinal herbs are more effective when applied as poultices or plasters. Many books provide precise directions on how best to prepare specific herbs. (See "Herbal Medicines" in the bibliography for a sampling of these books.) In this chapter, you will be introduced to the terminology and the most general of procedures so that you can feel at ease when the green revolution strikes you.

Precautions When Using Various Herbs

It is not possible to list all of the side effects and contraindications for the legion of herbs now being used. In cases of any glimmer of doubt, the reader is strongly advised to seek the advice of a knowledgeable health care giver. The following list touches upon some of the most frequently used herbs and warns of some of the most serious side effects:

Always read directions carefully, and in their absence seek a practical guide.

Some herbs are poisonous in high doses.

Those who suffer from chronic or serious illnesses should consult a health care practioner before using an herbal remedy.

Pregnant and nursing women should not use herbs without consulting a health care practitioner.

It is usually best to avoid giving any but well-tried and trusted herbs to children. Herbs are best avoided in children under the age of two. Consult your pediatrician.

People under the age of sixteen or over the age of sixty-five should approach herbs with caution. It is probably best for them to use reduced or diluted doses.

Generally speaking, it is always best to begin with the lowest recommended dose of an herb and increase it gradually if necessary.

The leaf of rhubarb is very poisonous. Ingestion can lead to severe kidney and liver damage.

The fruit of lily of the valley is considered very poisonous.

Sassafras, once used as a flavoring for root beer, has been banned for use as a flavoring for fifty years. Ingestion of the herb can interfere with liver enzymes.

Hellebore, monkshood, and larkspur are all poisonous and are not to be used internally.

The following herbs can be toxic and should not be used as home remedies: aconite, arnica, belladonna, bittersweet, calabar bean, camphor (internally), celandine (externally), daffodils, ergot, foxglove, hellebore, ignatius beans, jimsonweed, mandrake, mayflower, nux vomica, poison hemlock, saffron, spurge, squill, tobacco (internally), tonka beans, white bryony, and wormwood.

People with heart or blood pressure problems should avoid licorice root, gentian, and goldenseal.

Do not use alfalfa if you have an impaired immune system.

Do not use chamomile if you suffer from pollen-related allergies.

People who have a blood-clotting disorder or are taking anticlotting medicines, including aspirin, should avoid taking ginkgo biloba.

Dong quai should not be used by women who are menstruating.

Burdock taken internally can interfere with iron absorption.

Ground or powdered psyllium seeds, used to increase dietary fiber, can cause gas and stomach discomfort. Begin with less than the

smallest recommended dose and increase gradually so your system
can adjust. Be sure to drink at least eight glasses of water a day
when using this herb.

If you are taking any prescription or over-the-counter drugs, ask your
physician, herbalist, or pharmacist about possible interactions. Bear
in mind that these professionals may be uncertain about synthetic
drug and botanical or herbal interactions. Very little research is
available in this area.

If you experience nausea, itching, or diarrhea after using an herb, stop
taking it and consult a health care professional. You may be allergic
to the herb.

If you see no improvement of a minor condition after two weeks of
using an herb, consult your health care practitioner.

St. John's wort should not be taken in conjunction with any
antidepressant. This herb has unfavorable interactions with L-dopa,
used to treat Parkinson's disease, and tryptophan, an essential
amino acid. It should not be taken with foods that contain
tyramine, an amine found in some herbs, putrefied animal tissue,
and cheese. People who take St. John's wort will find they are
sensitive to light and may be prone to sunburn and sun rashes.

White willow bark contains salicin, the source of salicylic acid, which
is used in making aspirin. The bark has the same potential as
aspirin to irritate the stomach lining.

Some herbs should be used only in small quantities and with caution,
as they can have negative side effects. These include: bloodroot,
goldenseal, lobelia, rue, tansy, and valerian.

Recipes for Success

When preparing herbal remedies, there are several general rules of which
you should be aware. Always keep your herbs in tightly sealed containers.
Be aware that many herbs have uncertain shelf lives and can decompose
spontaneously, becoming ineffective with time. Be sure the utensils you
use are clean and your water is pure.

When you begin to read herbals, you will notice that the recipes for
some remedies are written in ounces, others are written in grams — the

primary unit of weight in the metric system — and still others are written in teaspoons. You can substitute 1 tablespoon or ½ ounce for 12 grams.

When measuring herbs do not use a teaspoon, as spoon sizes vary considerably from one set of flatware to another. Remember, too, that you cannot use a measuring cup to measure herbs. A measuring cup is used for liquid, not dry, measure.

Be aware that powdered herbs are more concentrated than fresh herbs; you need fewer of them than you do of fresh herbs.

Decoctions

Hard substances such as barks, roots, and twigs must be prepared with a great deal of heat to release their active principles.

1. Break the bark, roots, and twigs into small pieces.
2. Put 1 ounce of the herbs and 4 cups of water into a stainless steel or enamel pot.
3. Boil the water for about ten minutes, until the water content is reduced to approximately 3 cups.
4. Strain.
5. Decoctions may be stored in the refrigerator up to four days.
6. Doses are usually given in cups per day.

Electuaries

Sometimes, an herb is quite bitter; many herbalists believe this is important to the herb's therapeutic action (see page 184). However, some people cannot or will not swallow a bitter herb. In this case:

1. Measure the required dose of powdered herb.
2. Add enough honey, slippery elm, or coconut butter to make a paste. (Do not give honey to children under three years old.)
3. Roll the mix into a pill-sized ball.
4. Swallow the ball with juice.

Infusions

1. Bruise (lightly pound) 1 ounce of dried herbs in a clean cloth.

2. Pour 3 cups of boiling water (do not use reheated water) over the herb in a china, glass, crockery, or stainless steel vessel.
3. Cover the mixture tightly.
4. Let steep for twenty to thirty minutes.
5. Infusions may be stored in the refrigerator for up to four days.

Juice, Herbal

1. Wash the necessary amount of plant parts under cold, running water.
2. While the plant parts are still wet, place them in a juice extractor.
3. Immediately add the juice to tea or water.
4. If you have additional juice, put it in an airtight container and refrigerate.
5. Herb juice may be stored in the refrigerator for several days.

Pills

You can purchase herbal pills or prepare them at home. Some herbalists believe that herbal pills are less potent than liquids. They feel that the heat and water used in preparation help to release healing agents. Other herbalists contend it is important to experience the bitter taste of the herb because the bitterness provokes bodily reactions, such as the flow of bile and digestive juices. These functions can be useful in the treatment of various disorders such as gallbladder problems and gastrointestinal disturbances.

1. Steam hard roots to soften them.
2. Put enough water into a pot so it does not touch the bottom of your colander.
3. Bring the water to a boil and carefully place the colander into the pot.
4. Layer the herb parts in the colander.
5. Reduce heat to simmer and cover the pot until the herbs begin to appear wilted.
6. Put the herbs through a good quality coffee grinder to grind them into powder.
7. Blend in sufficient honey and arrowroot powder to form a thick paste. (Do not give honey to children under the age of three.)
8. Using your fingers, form small, firm, pea-sized balls.
9. Dry the balls in indirect sunlight or place them on a baking sheet and put them in the oven for a few minutes.

10. Store the pills in a dark-colored jar in a cool, dark place.

Raw Herbs

If hard herbs are to be consumed raw, they are normally ground into a powder and taken in capsules. This can be accomplished at home:

1. If the herbs are hard, such as red ginseng, they should first be steamed in order to soften them.
2. Put enough water into a pot so it will not touch the bottom of your colander.
3. Bring the water to a boil and carefully place the colander into the pot.
4. Layer the herb parts in the colander.
5. Reduce heat to simmer and cover the pot until the herbs begin to appear wilted.
6. Put the herbs through a good quality coffee grinder.
7. Powdered herbs should be stored in a jar in a dry, dark place. To preserve their potency, herbs should not be exposed to direct sunlight or excessive heat.

Teas

An herbal tea is basically a water extract that is usually prepared from the soft part of a plant — the leaves, whole herb, or flowers. Teas are a pleasant way to get your herbs, but commercially prepared herbal tea bags usually do not have medicinal doses of the active ingredients. If the active ingredients are not water soluble, you won't get any therapeutic benefit from drinking the tea.

Although tea is usually taken hot, some herbs lose their therapeutic value when warmed.

To prepare a cold tea:

1. Measure the recommended amount of herbs into a china, glass, crockery, or stainless steel vessel.
2. Cover the herbs with cold bottled or filtered water, and soak overnight.
3. Warm slightly if you wish and strain before drinking.

For hot tea:

1. Use only china, glass, crockery, or stainless steel vessels.

2. Pour 8 ounces of freshly boiled water over 1 heaping teaspoon of cut and sifted herbs or 1 level teaspoon of powdered herb. (If you are using encapsulated herbs, be aware that three to four capsules contain approximately one teaspoon of herb.)
3. Cover and let steep for at least five minutes.
4. Use a stainless steel or natural cloth strainer to strain the tea before drinking.

Tincture

1. Put 1 ounce of dried herb or 3 ounces of fresh herb in a small, sterile, airtight glass bottle.
2. Add a moderate amount of drinking alcohol; 100 proof rice wine or vodka is best.
3. Cork the bottle and put it in a warm spot (at least 70°F).
4. Shake the bottle twice each day for the next two to six weeks.
5. After two weeks, drops of the tincture may be added to water or tea. Tinctures may also be used in cool compresses.

Tonic Liqueurs

1. Place approximately 1 ounce of herbs in a quart of spirit. Rice wine is traditional but vodka or tequila may also be used.
2. Place the mixture in a dark place and allow it to sit for two to six weeks.
3. One or, at most, two sake-size cupfuls of the tonic liqueur may be consumed daily, usually after dinner or at bedtime.

Externally Applied Herbs

The external use of herbs is generally safe, but skin eruptions and rashes can occur.

Bath, Full

1. Cover approximately 7 ounces of dried herbs or 6 quarts of fresh herbs with cool water.
2. Soak the herbs overnight.
3. Heat the mixture.

4. Strain and add the liquid to a tub of water.
5. Sit in the bath for twenty minutes or so.

Bath, Sitz

1. Cover approximately 3 ounces of dried herbs or 2¹/₂ quarts of fresh herbs with cool water.
2. Soak the herbs overnight.
3. Heat the mixture.
4. Strain and add the liquid to a tub containing enough water to cover the area of your kidneys.

Essential Oils

These oils are responsible for the distinct flavor or odor of the plant from which they are obtained. They are used in the manufacture of perfumes and flavorings and are very popular as adjuncts to massage and for treating wounds. The whole field of aromatherapy revolves around essential or volatile oils.

Essential oils prepared for aromatherapy usage should be used diluted; they are quite concentrated and can irritate or even burn your skin if used undiluted. Internal use of standardized essential oils in delayed release capsules has emerged as a safe and valuable remedy. Examples are peppermint and fennel oil for the effective relief of digestive and bowel upsets.

1. Add 6 to 10 drops of an essential oil to 1 ounce of canola oil. Almond, apricot, or grapeseed oil can also be used; they are more expensive but impart additional luxury.
2. Shake well before using during a massage.
3. Add about 3 drops to a glass of water and use as a mouth, ear, or eyewash.

Fomentation

1. Prepare a hot tea (see page 185).
2. Soak a soft towel or cloth in the tea.
3. Remove the towel and wring slightly so it is wet but not dripping.
4. When the fomentation is as hot as you can tolerate, place it on the affected area.

5. Cover the wet cloth with a second, warm cloth to hold in the heat.
6. Repeat the above procedure as needed.

Ointment

1. Heat two cups of pure lard to 385° to 390° F.
2. Beware of spattering oil as you add 4 full handfuls of finely crumbled dry herbs or 6 full handfuls of chopped fresh herb parts.
3. Stir.
4. Wait one minute, remove from heat, cover.
5. Let the mixture stand overnight.
6. Heat gently until the mixture liquifies.
7. Stir in 4 tablespoons of virgin olive oil.
8. Squeeze through cheesecloth into a crockery or glass container.
9. Let stand till solidified.

Plaster

1. Prepare a steamed or pulped poultice (see the following preparations).
2. Place the herbs between two layers of material.
3. Place the plaster on the afflicted area. Plasters can be left in place for lengthy periods of time.

Caution: Plasters are normally prepared from rubefacient herbs that can redden and irritate the skin. Follow the directions carefully.

Poultice, Pulped

1. Place fresh plant material on a clean white cloth.
2. Fold so the herbs are inside the cloth.
3. Place a rolling pin on top of the cloth and roll to crush the herbs.
4. Place the poultice on the affected area and wrap with a second cloth to hold in body heat.

Poultice, Steamed

1. Put enough water into a pot so it will not touch the bottom of your colander.
2. Bring the water to a boil and carefully place the colander into the pot.
3. Layer the herb parts in the colander.

4. Reduce heat to simmer and cover the pot.
5. When the herbs have wilted and become soft, remove them from the colander.
6. Allow to cool for ten minutes.
7. Place the herbs on the affected area.
8. Fold a dish-towel-size cloth and wrap it around the affected area.
9. Remove when the poultice has cooled. Reapply as necessary.

Using Commercial Products

For the most part, it is no longer necessary to grow or prepare therapeutic herbs by yourself. Health food stores abound, and their shelves are fully stocked with commercially prepared tablets, capsules, and liquids.

Predictable health benefits can only be expected when one uses carefully prepared standardized and researched herbal extracts. There are many substandard herbal dietary supplements. Caveat emptor.

In Western society, there have been increasing attempts to standardize herbal products so that they can be used in forms that produce a reasonably consistent biological effect. Herbal products are not essential nutrients, and they do not have recommended dietary allowances. Therefore, "dosages" of herbs are often a best guess unless a standardized herbal extract is used. Even standardization of an herbal extract does not always permit accurate dosing information to be given because, in many cases, dose response studies have not been performed.

The authors recommend that consumers purchase herbal products from reputable purveyors of dietary supplements that produce standardized extracts from herbs and botanicals. If a product does not have evidence of standardized contents or clearly labeled supporting data from the manufacturer, the authors recommend that the reader not use the product.

You can also purchase fresh and dried herbs at health food stores and herb shops. When purchasing herbs, remember that both fresh and dried herbs should be stored in airtight containers that prevent light from entering.

Herbal products frequently have a short shelf life, losing potency as time passes. For an herb to be fully active, it frequently must be less than six months old. However, to ensure that the dose you get is consistent, buy herbs that contain standardized extracts. These are most likely to be in tablet or capsule form.

To produce tablets, powdered botanicals are mixed with flowing, binding, and disintegration agents before being pressed into the desired form. Today, the caplet shape is quite popular and is a very convenient way to get your herbs. The processing, however, reduces assimilation of the active ingredients and during processing the herb is mixed with adulterants. Although quite safe, the presence of binding agents does increase the risk of allergic reactions. A process called the quadgyric method involves preparing a mild extract in which the liquid is evaporated, the residue is granulated, ground, and made into a tablet. The process is less likely to cause an allergic reaction. In addition, herbs prepared this way are more easily assimilated.

Herbs are also sold in a form known as tincture. Tinctures are prepared by soaking an herb in alcohol. Usually, the ratio is 1 part herb to 2 to 10 parts alcohol. Tinctures are usually marketed in a bottle with an eyedropper in the lid. Fluid extracts are similar to tinctures, but they are more concentrated. It is best to avoid these products if you wish to avoid alcohol.

In another process called spagyric, the material left after production of the tincture is burned and the marc is reintroduced to the tincture as a soluble material. These liquid products are easily absorbed, but are sometimes unpleasant tasting.

Some adults may believe that "the worse it tastes, the better it is for you." Children may, however, require a different motivation. They can usually be coaxed into taking the liquid if you offer them a cookie or favorite drink immediately afterward. You can also try preparing an electuary (see page 183). Children may actually be eager to try a preparation if they can participate in making it.

Herbal products may also be purchased as dry extracts (*extracts sicca*). After the liquid extract is prepared, the fluid is removed through techniques such as freeze-drying. Because dry extracts readily attract moisture, they should be ground and kept in airtight containers. In an oily drug extract (*olea medicata*), oil-soluble active ingredients are extracted when they are macerated in an oil such as peanut, olive, or almond. Because the extract is not stable, the product must be used immediately after opening. Sometimes, oily drug extracts are encapsulated in soft gel.

No matter what preparation you buy, read the labels carefully to be sure that the amount of active ingredient duplicates the dosage you are supposed to have. Be sure to carefully follow directions regarding dosage and safety. It is probably best to avoid products that contain more than two or three active ingredients. The more ingredients, the lower will be the dose of each. In addition, you cannot be sure that the company has adequately researched interactions between the ingredients.

Using Traditional Chinese Herbs

Although anyone can whip up a cup of tea, the use of traditional Chinese herbs requires a bit more knowledge. Some Chinese herbs can be made into tea or even soup. Some are simply chewed. Sometimes, alcohol-based tonics are prepared. Complications arise because Chinese herbalists rarely use herbs singly; they are almost always compounded. Compounding of herbs relies upon the laws of yin and yang, the action of individual herbs, and the fundamental principles of Chinese medicine.

Herbs may be yang—warming the body and increasing physiological activity— or yin—cooling the body by sedating excessive physiological activity. Some herbs affect the internal regions of the body, or viscera, and are therefore yin, while others "float"; their reactions occur on the surface of the body in the muscle and skin. Warm and cool herbs have a relatively gentle effect compared to hot and cold herbs. For example, herbs that contain essential oils are considered spicy cool. Today's biochemists understand this to mean that essential oils can dilate peripheral blood vessels in and below the skin and membranes, causing the surface to warm while cooling the interior.

It is best to use cool, mild, and warm herbs at first. Once you have gained experience, you can explore hot and cold ones, which should always be used sparingly in comparison to less extreme herbs. When hot or cold herbs are used, they must be balanced in a formula containing other herbs so that the result is no more extreme than warm or cool. The herbs will still have a powerful effect, but the formula will not shock the body with extreme energy.

Traditionally, Chinese herbs are compounded according to the Four Responsible Positions formula. There are four positions in a formula: king, minister, assistant, and servant. The king is the principal herb. It is usually a powerful herb that has tonic or energizing effects as well as a specific action. Ginseng is often used as the king herb. A second herb, known as the minister, reinforces the king's actions. The minister has a similar action to the king but may enter different meridians to balance the formula's energy.

The third position is occupied by the assistant. This herb counteracts any undesirable actions that may be precipitated by the king or minister, or tones up qualities that the other herbs do not. The assistant brings harmony and balance to the mixture. The servant occupies the fourth position and harmonizes the other ingredients to ensure proper absorption. Sometimes, the servant's role is to provide quick systematic relief, such as an end to pain.

Consider one such formula composed of ginseng, atractylus, ginger, and licorice. Ginseng is the king; it tones up the spleen and increases production of essential energy. Atractylus is the minister. A tonic or energizing herb, it also tones the spleen, adds energy, and regulates fluid balance and appetite.

The assistant is ginger, which supports the king by warming the intestines and improving circulation. If circulation were blocked, the effects of the ginseng might be too concentrated in a particular area rather than being distributed throughout the body. Licorice root is the servant, enhancing the absorption of the other herbs and acting as a tonic to the stomach, lungs, and kidney. It is also a detoxifier that rids both the body and the herbal compound of any toxins, thus preventing negative side effects.

Traditional Chinese medicine includes the use of herbs and botanicals that can now be purchased in standardized extracts from industry leaders in dietary supplement manufacture. This field includes the Allergy Research Group of San Leandro, California, BioTherapies, Inc., of Fairfield, New Jersey, and Nature's Way of Springville, Utah. Considering the complexity of the art, if you wish to use Chinese herbs, commercial preparations are probably your best bet. These are almost always accompanied by helpful instructions. In addition to their ease of use, commercial preparations usually cost less than homemade formulas. The availability of these preparations means you have access to them whenever you need them and for as long as necessary.

You may purchase herbs as extracts. The energy and blood tonic *shou wu chih* is sold in this form. People use this preparation to help them sleep soundly and to increase their sexual energy. Readily available, too, are extracts of the popular *Panax ginseng*. Because water (aqueous) extracts provide a perfect environment for the growth of microorganisms, such products must be put into airtight vials immediately after manufacturing. Chinese herbal liquids are usually bottled in 10 cc ampules and sold in boxes of ten.

To preserve the sterility of the contents, the vials are sliced with a glass-cutting stone that is included in the package. A plastic safety cap found in the box is then fitted over the ampule and the ampule's head is snapped off. The extract is drunk through a small straw. One of the most popular of these products is Peking royal jelly oral liquid. Royal jelly, secreted by worker bees, is the food of queen bees. Because queen bees live about twenty times longer than other bees in the hive, the jelly has been investigated as a perfect food. Royal jelly contains virtually every vitamin, mineral, essential amino acid, and many female hormones. It is believed to be both energizing and fertility producing. In addition to the jelly, Peking royal jelly oral liquid consists of herbs and is considered a supertonic.

Chinese herbal products are also available as pills or tablets. Halonyuan, or black dragon tonic pill, is a much-revered tonic, a preparation believed to increase strength and energy. It combines several tonics with ginseng and deer antler extract and is believed to promote health and generate vitality. Four ginseng dragon eggs is an extremely potent tonic containing four varieties of ginseng and twenty-six other tonic herbs.

Literature about Chinese herbs is traditionally arranged according to their therapeutic effects. A Chinese pharmacopoeia will be divided into categories such as diaphoretics, digestives, tonics, and so forth. (See the section on herbal terminology beginning on p. 153.)

When preparing *Andrographis paniculata* for use as a medicinal, people boil one to three handfuls of fresh leaf and drink the "tea" three times a day, before meals. Some people grind dried leaves to a powder and formulate a .8 cm (approximately three-tenths of an inch) pill using honey as a binder. They take three to six of these pills three to four times daily, usually before meals and at bedtime. Commercially prepared capsules are now available and are sold in 250 and 500 mg sizes, as marked on the label. Depending on the size of the capsule, people take either four or two capsules, two or three times a day before meals. Users are cautioned that the preparations may cause vomiting.

Ayurvedic Herbs

To obtain the herbs or teas used in Ayurvedic medicine, contact:

Ancient Healing Ways
Route 3, Box 259
Espanola, NM 87532
(800) 359-2940

BioTherapies, Inc.
9 Commerce Rd.
Fairfield, NJ 07004
(800) 700-7325

Maharashi Ayur-Ved Products, Inc.
P.O. Box 49667
Colorado Springs, CO 80949
(800) 255-8332

The Tea Garden Herbal Emporium
903 Colorado Ave. Suite 200
Santa Monica, CA 90401
(310) 205-0104

No matter what kind of herbal product you purchase, you must put your faith in the manufacturer. Happily, today's food supplement industry is far more scientifically grounded than it has ever been. The Natural Products Quality Assurance Council and the National Natural Foods Association are working to create industry-wide standards of quality control. Unfortunately, it can still be difficult for the consumer to sort fact from fiction. Each manufacturer claims its product is superior and has the highest possible quality control. However, chemical analysis often reveals that the product is not what it claims to be. Additives or fillers are often used because a product is cheaper to manufacture that way, but fillers can reduce the effectiveness of the active component. Ultimately, you are your own best watchdog.

You must do your homework: Ask pharmacists and health care providers which companies they trust; check newspaper indices to see information about the company. The Office of Alternative Medicine is promising to produce a long overdue register of effective remedies of natural origin. You might also send for the free FDA publication "Choosing Medical Treatments." Write to the Consumer Information Center, Pueblo, Colorado 81009 and request item 537. If you would like to work with a trained herbalist, you can obtain a referral by writing to the Institute for Traditional Medicine, 2017 S.E. Hawthorne Blvd., Portland, Oregon 97014.

To obtain information on a particular herb, contact the Herb Research Foundation, 1007 Pearl Street Suite 200, Boulder, Colorado 80302; telephone: (303) 449-2265, fax (303) 449-7849. For 75 cents per reference, you can obtain information on specific products from Natural Products Alert (NAPRALERT) at the College of Pharmacy–UIC, 833 S. Wood Street, Chicago, IL 60612; (312) 996-2246.

Several books on herbal medicine are available from the Wild Rose College of Natural Healing, 1745 W. 4th Avenue, Vancouver, B.C., V6J 1M2; telephone (604) 734-4596, fax (604) 734-4597.

You might consider subscribing to:

Health Consciousness: An Holistic Magazine
P.O. Box 550
Oviedo, FL 32765
(407) 365-6681

Health Freedom News (a magazine about natural preventive medicine)
212 West Foothill Blvd.
P.O. Box 688
Monrovia CA 91017
(818) 357-2181

Nutriceutical News International
75 Plymouth St.
Fairfield, NJ 07004
Fax: (201) 276-0639

Townsend Letter for Doctors (a newsletter focusing on alternative health and holistic medicine)
911 Tyler St.

Pt. Townsend, WA 98368
(360) 385-6021

A great deal of information is available through computerized databases and on-line services such as America Online and WorldNet. MEDLINE, a centralized database, provides access to a vast amount of health and pharmaceutical information. Mapis, which originates in New Delhi, India, provides information on medicinal plants from six hundred journals. Various software programs provide easy access to information on a variety of herbal medicines. Discs for both IBM and Mac systems are available from: P.O. Box 873, Ben Lomond, CA 95005; telephone: (408) 336-2442.

Interactive BodyMind Information System (IBIS) is another software program that provides information on Chinese herbs and other botanicals as well as on various types of alternative medicine. Some dietary supplement companies have invested a great deal of money in consumer education. One company, BioTherapies, Inc., has a consumer education service and a newsletter on the Internet at WWW.biotherapies.com. Remember, if you are seriously ill, consult a health care practitioner. Trying to self-medicate an illness may prove to be grave folly.

Sources of Herbs and Herbal Products

Check your local Yellow Pages to locate herb distributors in your area. These retailers may be able to provide information on mail-order sources. You might also contact the following companies:

Biotherapies, Inc.
9 Commerce Rd.
Fairfield, NJ 07004
(800) 700-7325

Companion Plants
7247 N. Coolville Ridge Rd.
Athens, OH 45701
(614) 592-65643

Crystal Star Herbal Nutrition
14409 Cuesta Ct.
Sonora, CA 95370
(209) 532-6474

Dragon River Herbal
P.O. Box 74
Highway 285
Ojo Caliente, NM 87549
(505) 583-2118

Eclectic Institute
14385 S.E. Lusted Rd.
Sandy, OR 97055
(503) 668-3227

Frontier Cooperative Herbs
3021 78th St.
Norway, IA 52318
(800) 786-1388

Health Concerns
2415 Mariner Square Dr. #3
Alameda, CA 94501
(800) 233-9355

Herb and Spice Collection
P.O. Box 118
Norway, IA 52318
(800) 365-4372

HerbPharm's Whole Herb Catalog
P.O. Box 116
Williams, OR 97544
(503) 846-6262

K'an Herb Company
6001 Butler Lane
Scotts Valley, CA 95066
(408) 438-9450
Fax: (408) 438-9457

Kanpo Formulas
P.O. Box 60279
Sacramento, CA 95860
(916) 487-9044

Mayway Trading Company
780 Broadway
San Francisco, CA 95073
(415) 788-3646

Natural Resources
6680 Harvard Dr.
Sebastopol, CA 95472
(707) 747-0390

Nature's Herb Company
1010 46th St.
Emeryville, CA 94608
(510) 601-0700

Nature's Way
10 Mountain Springs Pkwy.
Springville, UT 84663
(801) 489-1500
Fax: (801) 489-1700

NutriLife
605 E. San Antonio St.
Victoria, Texas 77901
(800) 742-7513

Penn Herb Company, Ltd.
10601 Decatur Rd., Suite 2
Philadelphia, PA 19154
(800) 523-9971
Fax: (215) 632-7945

Pharmanex
625 Cochran St.
Simi Valley, CA 93065
(800) 999-6229

Rainbow Light
207 McPherson St.
Department P
Santa Cruz, CA 95060
(800) 635-1233

Rosemary House
120 S. Market St.
Mechanicsburg, PA 17055
(717) 697-5111

Twinlab
2120 Smithtown Ave.
Ronkonkoma, NY 11779
(516) 467-3140

Seelect Herb Tea Company
P.O. Box 1969
Camarillo, CA 93011
(805) 484-0899

Conclusion

The use of herbs in the treatment of disease is a long and noble tradition. Herbalists have been counted among the most revered members of society. Today, you can partake of the wisdom of the ages.

Scientists today are learning more and more about the potential efficacy and possible dangers of nutriceuticals. Therefore, herbal use today is safer and more dependable than it has ever been. So whether you like to hold a warm cup of fragrant tea in your hands, pop a pill with a swig of water, or drink a potent potion, the world of herbal medicines has something for you.

Conclusion

From shaman to radiologist, the story of medical history is almost as long as civilization itself. It is a story of struggle against disease, ignorance, and inflexibility. It is also a story of conflict between physicians and pharmacists, establishment medicine and alternatives, innovators and bureaucrats.

One of the basic conflicts has revolved around the very nature of disease. Although traditional Chinese medicine has always believed that internal balance is the root of health and imbalance the root of disease, in the Western world establishment medicine has steadily turned away from those concepts. Some practitioners of allopathic medicine have advocated doing the least, letting nature run its course, helping the body only when necessary.

Others believe that man can control nature. They have recommended treatments that are faster and more efficient than the body's defenses. Some have advocated the use of synthetic pharmaceuticals, others surgery. Even these two camps have often been at loggerheads with each other. For example, in seventeenth-century France the king's physician said, "The great abuse of medicine is due to the multiplicity of useless remedies and the neglect of bloodletting." Now, even bloodletting has found a place in modern medicine with the amazing use of leeches in severe injuries and poorly healing wounds.

Surgeon and pharmacist do, however, have one thing in common: Both believe themselves to be "men of science." Unfortunately, in many cases, modern men of science seem to have found science and nature to be incompatible. To these men, natural options are inefficient, archaic, or just plain superstitious. These stubborn practitioners will not survive the increasing demand for natural options or the increasing self-reliance of the health care consumer in the next millennium.

In the hands of establishment medicine, germ theory, synthetic medicine, and big business worked together to wrest control of the body away from the individual. People have become increasingly dissatisfied with the solutions offered by the "establishment." Many have turned back to earlier pursuits. We have, in fact, come full circle. Mankind spent most of its history using herbal medicines. We then spent a generation or more creating synthetics to mimic nature. In recent years, we have been preoccupied with the effect of synthetic drugs on humankind. The biotechnology developed primarily for the pursuit of synthetic remedies is now being used to return us to our beginnings. Modern man, like our old friend Paracelsus, is beginning to believe that Mother Nature has answers to most, if not all the plagues of society.

Nature Will Provide

Nature's answers lie in the system of balance that we see all around us. Consider, for instance, homeostasis — the state of equilibrium in the body. Homeostasis maintains balance in various functions and in the chemical compositions of fluids and tissues. Physiological and biochemical actions within each organism return that organism to "normal" conditions. To maintain normal body temperature, the body perspires and cools down or generates goose pimples and shivers to warm up. When people are diseased or stressed or very old or very young, balance cannot be achieved as quickly.

In addition, a lack of balance indicates a disease state. If, for example, a person eats a meal high in sugar, the tendency is for blood glucose to rise to high levels, but a healthy or normal body has the capability of regulating the glucose concentration so it returns to normal levels. When a person is diabetic, this ability is impaired; the glucose remains at higher levels for much longer periods.

Nature has provided a system of balance by which a person or a living thing can heal itself — up to a point. There is a limit beyond which healing cannot occur or is incomplete — that is when the Paracelsian concept of the "external physician" comes into play. Many scientists today believe that the Earth is also a living organism that experiences balance. Nature's system of balance permits the Earth to heal itself according to what is termed the Gaia principle, named for the Greek goddess who became the mother of the

Titans and the Cyclopes — the Earth Mother. Some of the best examples of the Earth Mother's protective system can be found in the plant kingdom.

More than twenty-five thousand species of flowering plants share the planet with men and animals, yet to a plant, almost every single organism in the animal world represents a predator. In the rain forest, where the number of predators is practically incalcuable, plants have many chemicals that help protect them. Some protection comes in the form of odors, colors, and textures that repel animals; other forms include chemicals that can bring about the healing of an injured plant or the death of a plant predator. A multitude of phytochemicals play a role in the physiology, reproduction, and protection of both plants and animals.

According to Christopher Joyce, author of *Earthly Goods: Medicine Hunting in the Rainforest,* "As scientists have peeled back the chemical layers of tropical life, they have discovered extraordinary substances — tree saps that kill viruses, seaweed that blocks cancer, spider poisons that combat neurological disease, even secretions from frogs that could treat depression and stroke."

A similar story is told in *Bombardier Beetles and Fever Trees: A Close-up Look at Chemical Warfare and Signals in Animals and Plants.* Written by William Agosta, a professor of chemistry and head of the Laboratory of Organic Chemistry at Rockefeller University in New York City, the book examines chemicals that play a role in the lifestyles of plants and insects. In reviewing the book, Murray Blum, a research professor of entomology at the University of Georgia, writes, "Agosta clearly believes that these compounds may offer a solution to many of the problems that plague our planet. Certainly, these chemicals constitute important medicinals against cancer and are a critical source of life-saving antibiotics. Beyond that, the author believes that the availability of biologically active natural chemicals in rain forests may inhibit the indiscriminate clearing of these habitats."

In the 1980s, people became aware that the rain forests were diminishing — rapidly. Large expanses of the forests are disappearing because of a slash-and-burn philosophy, in which acres of land are burned each year to create fields for planting and pastures for cattle grazing. The rain forests are also being destroyed by logging. Even with public awareness of these problems, it is predicted that more than half of the rain forests will have vanished in less than four decades. What will become of the wildlife that teems within these jungles? Currently, one-half a percent of the species in these forests disappear from the planet each year.

In the mid 1980s, cancer and AIDS researchers as well as indigenous populations banded together in the belief that the rain forest can be saved because within it grow cures for a host of diseases. Pharmaceutical companies began to realize that the rain forest might harbor effective drugs. Today, ethnobotonists, anthropologists, cancer researchers, loggers, businessmen, ecologists, and conservationists swarm in and out of the forests, united by a common goal: to preserve the forests by proving that it is more profitable to sustain them and the products they yield than to get a quick return on investments by cutting the forests down.

The reestablishment of a man-nature team may restore balance and health to Earth and its inhabitants, but restoration of harmony does not require that we abandon the trappings of modern society. We know modern technology will play a vital role in bringing health to the planet.

Technology that can reveal how, when, and why biochemical messages are carried to and "turn on" cellular particles will help us find the answers that nature holds. The therapeutic efficacy of various herbs is already being demonstrated by the modern scientific methodology called signal transduction technology. In studies using this technology, concentrates from *Andrographis paniculata* were shown to have very specific effects on the transfer of cellular messages. This research has centered around certain enzymes that play a vital role in coordinating the process of cell proliferation, which is at the heart of cancer and other diseases. The ability to see inside of cells will radically alter the use of natural medicines and result in an herbal revolution.

The Miracle Herbs

Herbs can work wonders. They can provide cures without many of the debilitating side effects commonly associated with synthetic drugs. AIDS, cancer, heart diseases, and the common cold may be cured by any one of a number of herbs currently being investigated. With the aid of signal transduction technology, firm scientific evidence will substantiate the claims made for the therapeutic value of natural agents. Opposition from physicians, scientists, and government agencies should fly in the face of this overwhelming evidence.

By providing cures for previously incurable diseases, herbs may even provide a "cure" for the ailments of the planet. In our newfound appreciation of all things green, perhaps we will learn to cherish and protect this small green planet and all its inhabitants — and wouldn't that be a miracle for herbs?

Glossary

Alchemist   Practitioner of the ancient chemistry known as alchemy.

Alchemy   A philosophical and medical tradition central to scientific research in ancient civilizations; the medieval version of chemistry whose underlying idea is a belief in transmutation.

Alkali   A metal whose water solution is bitter, slippery, caustic, and basic rather than acidic.

Alkaline   Having the properties of an alkali.

Alkaloids   Crystalline plant products whose molecules contain carbon, hydrogen, nitrogen and oxygen; usually the active principle of a crude drug. Many, such as morphine, have physiological action.

Allopathic   Modern conventional Western medicine; related to that method of treating disease using remedies that produce effects different from those caused by the disease.

Anabolism   The process by which nutritive matter is assimilated and converted into living substance.

Andrographolide   An active bitter principle of the *Andrographis paniculata* leaf. Four of these colorless, crystalline substances constitute up to 2 percent by dry weight of the herb's leaves.

Angina   Spasmodic attacks of suffocating chest pain.

Angiogenesis   Development of new blood vessels.

Angiography   X-ray examination following injection of radio-opaque substances.

Anorexia   Loss of appetite, particularly when associated with a disease.

Antibodies   The basis of immunity: proteins produced in the blood in response to an antigen; they destroy or weaken bacteria and organic poisons.

Antigen   Substances such as bacteria, toxins, and foreign blood cells that stimulate production of an antibody.

Antioxidant   Substance that prevents oxidation, the process by which oxygen reacts with another chemical; they prevent the damage caused when high-energy oxygen produces radicals.

Antithrombolytic   Preventing a thrombus from dissolving.

Apoptosis   Programmed cell death.

Archipelago   Large group of islands.

Arteriosclerosis   A chronic disease characterized by impaired blood circulation that results from the hardening and thickening of arterial walls.

Atherosclerosis   A form of arteriosclerosis in which plaque containing cholesterol and lipids is deposited on the innermost layer of artery walls.

Atropine   An alkaloid derived from plants; used to dilate the pupils of the eyes and as an antispasmodic.

Ayurvedic   The ancient Indian practice of medicine, based on the Ayurveda, a comprehensive medical text written around 700 B.C.

Benign prostate hyperplasia   An abnormal increase in the size of the prostate, often referred to as BPH.

Biotechnology   The use of microorganisms or biological substances to perform industrial or manufacturing processes.

Capillaries   Minute vessels that connect arterioles and venules.

Catabolism   A process within the body by which complex chemical compounds break down into simpler ones, often accompanied by the release of energy.

Catalyst   A substance that accelerates a chemical reaction without being used up or altered by that reaction.

CD4   A molecule on the surface of a living cell to which HIV binds or attaches, thereby infecting the cell.

Chemotherapy   The use of chemical agents or drugs to treat diseases.

Collagen   A protein that is the main constituent of skin.

Complementary medicine   A branch of medicine in which nonallopathic techniques are used to enhance or complete the practice of medicine.

Congestive heart failure   The heart's inability to pump blood at sufficient pressure.

Cyclins   Proteins named for their cyclical appearance.

Cyclotron   A particle accelerator.

Cytokines   Molecules of hormones and hormonelike proteins that affect physiological processes at the cellular level by inducing activity in cells.

Cytoplasm   The semifluid substance outside the nucleus of a cell.

Cytotoxic   Poisonous to cells; most cancer treatments are cytotoxic — poisonous to rapidly reproducing cells while leaving normal cells unharmed.

Decoction   A concentrate formed by boiling down an herb in water.

Dexfenfluramine   An antiobesity drug sold under the brand name Redux; in combination with phentermine, the preparation is called Fen-Phen; the manufacturer withdrew dexfenfluramine from the market in September 1997.

Dilation   The act of expanding.

Dioscorein   Dried yam root.

DNA   Deoxyribonucleic acid; a large molecule of nucleic acid that carries genetic information; found primarily in chromosomes.

Dropsy   The name once used to indicate the medical condition now called edema.

Edema A condition characterized by an abnormal accumulation of fluid; usually caused by the heart's inability to pump blood at sufficient pressure, a condition known as congestive heart failure.

Embolism Obstruction or occlusion of a blood vessel by a mass such as a detached blood clot, foreign body, or air bubble.

Endorphins Naturally occurring opiates.

Endothelial cells Cells that make up the walls of blood vessels.

Endothelium A layer of epithelial cells lining serous cavities and vessels.

Enzyme Protein catalysts that slow down or speed up chemical reactions in our body.

Epidemiologist One who studies the causes, distribution, and control of disease within populations.

Epithelium Membranous tissue composed of one or several layers of cells that have little intercellular substances; forms the covering of most body surfaces and organs.

Ethnobotany The study of the plant lore and agricultural customs of a particular people.

Fenfluramine An antiobesity drug sold under the brand name Pondimin. It is half of the controversial weight control medication known as fen-phen. Fenfluramine was withdrawn from the market in September 1997.

Fen-phen A controversial antiobesity drug implicated in cases of heart valve damage. Fen-phen is a combination of dexfenfluramine and fenfluramine; all three were withdrawn from the market in September 1997.

Fibrin A protein that forms a fibrous network in the coagulation of blood.

Free radicals Atoms or groups of atoms that have at least one unpaired electron, which makes them highly reactive; cause oxidation to occur.

Genetic engineering A technology that permits researchers to develop organisms or cells whose offspring have genetic combinations that were not present in the parents.

Genome A complete set of chromosomes with the associated genes.

Glycosides These organic compounds occur abundantly in plants, where they have important regulatory, protective, and sanitary functions. Many compounds in this group have physiological effects on humans.

Hemoglobin The portion of red blood cells in vertebrates that contains the pigment and iron.

Hemostasis The stoppage of blood flow.

Histology The study of normal and diseased cells.

Homeopathy Treatment of disease through the administration of minute doses of a substance that in larger amounts produces disease symptoms.

Homeostasis An organism's or cell's ability to maintain internal equilibrium through the adjustment of physiological processes.

Hormones   Proteins produced in one tissue that travel via the bloodstream to another tissue, where they bring about such physiological activities as growth or metabolism.

Hypertension   High blood pressure.

Immunology   A branch of science concerned with the structure and function of the immune system, natural and acquired immunity, and laboratory techniques involving the interaction of antigens and antibodies.

In vitro   In an artificial environment outside a living organism.

In vivo   Within living organisms.

Infarction   Tissue death due to lack of oxygen.

Intraperitoneal   Relating to the inside of the fluid-producing sac consisting of a thin layer of epithelium and a thin layer of connective tissue that lines the abdominal cavity.

Ischemia   Decreased blood supply caused by constriction or obstruction of blood vessels.

Isoflavones   Natural estrogens of plant origin.

Kilogram   Metric measurement equivalent to 2.2 pounds.

Kinase   Any of various enzymes that facilitate the transfer of a phosphate group from a donor to a receptor.

Leukocytes   Colorless or white blood cells that protect the body from infection and disease. Also called white blood cells, white cells, and white corpuscles.

Life zone   Unique areas of habitat and climate, each zone is related to a particular geographical feature, such as a mountain slope, riverbank, or savannah.

Lipids   Organic water-insoluble fats, oils, sterols, and triglycerides that, along with proteins and carbohydrates, are the principal structural material of living cells.

Lymphoma   Malignant tumors in the lymph nodes or other lymphoid tissue.

Malignant   Runaway growth that chokes normal tissues.

Mechanism of action   Precise chemical and biological activity that produces desirable and predictable results.

Metabolism   The sum of processes governing the breakdown and synthesis of nutrients to generate energy and maintain life.

Microbiology   The biology of microorganisms and their effects on other living organisms.

Mitogen   An agent that brings about cell division.

Mitosis   A process in cell division in which the nucleus divides, resulting in two new nuclei. Each of the new nuclei contains a complete copy of the parent's chromosomes.

Monoclonals   Specific antibodies that the body can use as weapons against foreign invaders and cancerous growths.

Mutator genes   This class of genes normally protects the genes that are involved in cell division; protects them from undergoing mutation.

Myocardial   Pertaining to the myocardium.

Myocardial infarction   Necrosis of a region of the heart muscle caused by an interruption in the blood supply

Myocardium   Muscle tissue in the heart.

Necrosis   Death of tissue in living organisms.

Neuro-muscular-skeletal system   The interactions between nerves, muscles, and bones.

Nongenotoxic   Carcinogens that do not damage DNA.

Nutriceuticals   Naturally occurring agents that exert a positive influence in the human body.

Oncogenes   These genes prompt normal cell division; they give cells the signal to divide. When damaged or mutated, oncogenes cause their host cells to divide uncontrollably.

Oncology   The branch of medicine dealing with cancer.

Organelles   Components within cells.

Paracetamol   The British equivalent of acetaminophen.

Pathogen   A disease-causing agent, particularly a microorganism.

Pathology   The scientific study of the causes, processes, development, and consequences of diseases.

Phagocytosis   The process by which cells ingest and digest bacteria and other foreign particles.

Pharmacognosist   An expert in the medicinal uses of herbs.

Pharmacology   The study of the changes produced in people and animals through the use of chemical substances.

Pharmacopoeia   A book listing medicinal drugs and containing articles on their use; a collection of drugs.

Phosphorylation   The addition of a phosphate group to a molecule.

Phytochemicals   Chemicals found in plants.

Platelets   Very small bodies found in a mammal's blood plasma; promote blood clotting.

Pondimin   An antiobesity drug, the generic version of which is fenfluramine; half of the controversial weight control medication known as fen-phen; its manufacturer withdrew Pondimin from the market in September 1997.

Probiotics   Friendly bacteria.

Prophylactic   Tending to prevent a disease.

Prostatectomy   Removal of all or part of the prostate gland.

Protease inhibitor   A substance that halts the breakdown of enzymes that catalyze the breakdown of proteins by water.

Rain forest Dense tropical evergreen forest with an annual rainfall of at least one hundred inches.

Restenosis An overall decrease in the diameter of a blood vessel that had been previously constricted; it occurs after angioplasty due to a natural physiological process.

Sarcoma A malignant tumor in connective tissue.

Shaman Medicine man, witch doctor, or healer.

Signal transduction The passage of information to cellular particles. This information controls the cell cycle, turning various functions on and off.

Sonogram A diagnostic tool in which an image is made of the body through the use of transmitted and reflected sound waves.

Stenosis Narrowing of a duct or passage; stricture.

Strychnine An alkaloid derived from plants; used as a rodent poison and central nervous system stimulant.

Systolic pressure Rhythmic heart contractions that drive blood through the aorta and pulmonary artery after each dilation or diastole.

Thrombin An enzyme in blood that facilitates blood clotting; reacts with the protein fibrinogen to form fibrin, an elastic and insoluble protein that forms a network of fibers which coagulates blood.

Thromboembolism A blood vessel blockage caused by a blood clot that has become dislodged from its place of origin.

Thrombus Fibrinous clot formed in a blood vessel or heart cavity; may or may not be occlusive.

Topical Pertaining to the surface of the body.

Transmutation The central belief in alchemy; substances' energies can be purified so that they can be manipulated to create an enhanced physical substance (i.e., an herbal remedy or gold).

Tumor New tissue that develops from cells growing in an uncontrolled manner.

Tumor suppressor gene A type of gene that keeps new cell production at a moderate rate.

Volatile oils Rapidly evaporating, odorous oils that do not leave a greasy stain; found in various plant parts, depending on the particular family of plants. Frequently associated with fertilization or protection in plants, volatile oils act as hormones, regulators, and catalysts.

References

AIDS

Cohen, Jon. "PCR Patent Tangle Slows Quick Assay of HIV Levels." *Science,* June 6, 1997, p. 1488+.

_____. "AIDS: Advances Painted in Shades of Gray at a D.C. Conference." *Science,* January 31, 1997, pp. 615–16.

Edkins, Linda. "Gen-Probe Tackles HIV Screening Task." *Medical Herald,* February 1977, p. 45.

Golden, Arnold. "New AIDS Drugs Make PhRMA Optimistic." *Medical Herald,* February 1997, p. 47.

Hyde, Margaret O., and Forsyth, Elizabeth H., M.D. *AIDS: What Does It Mean to You?* New York: Walker and Co., 1992.

Rawls, Rebecca. "Peptidomimetic Molecules Show Biological Activity Against Cancer, AIDS." *Chemical and Engineering News,* April 8, 1996, pp. 37–39.

Reynolds, Jeffrey L. "Calm About AIDS Can Be Deceiving." *Newsday,* August 5, 1997, pp. A29+.

Sardi, Bill. "Can Cancer-Fighting Natural Products Combat Aids?" *Nutrition Science News,* March 1997, pp. 144–47.

Alternative Medicine

Baker, Beth. "The Mind-Body Connection: Putting the 'Faith Factor' to Work." *AARP Bulletin,* July/August 1997, p. 20.

Balch, James F., M.D., and Balch, Phyllis A., C.N.C. *Prescription for Nutritional Healing.* Garden City Park, N.Y.: Avery Publishing Group, 1990.

Boughton, Barbara. "The Healing Arts." *Modern Maturity,* September/October 1996, p. 70.

Bricklin, Mark. *The Practical Encyclopedia of Natural Healing.* Emmaus, Penn.: Rodale Press, 1976.

Carper, Jean. *Miracle Cures.* New York: HarperCollins, 1997.

"Health Watch: Alternative Services." *Newsday,* September 16, 1997, p. C9.

"Homeopathic Remedies." *Consumer Reports,* January 1987, pp. 60–62.

Lane, William I., and Comac, Linda. *Sharks Don't Get Cancer.* Garden City Park, N.Y.: Avery Publishing Group, 1992.

_____. *Sharks Still Don't Get Cancer.* Garden City Park, N.Y.: Avery Publishing Group, 1996.

Whitaker, Julian, M.D. *Dr. Whitaker's Guide to Natural Healing.* Rocklin, Calif.: Prima Publishing, 1994.

Wilk, Dr. Chester A. *Medicine, Monopolies, and Malice.* Garden City Park, N.Y.: Avery Publishing Group, 1996.

Yap, Leslie. "Avoiding the Allure." *Modern Maturity*, September/October 1996, p. 69.

Andrographis paniculata

Akbarsha, M. A.; Manivannan, B.; Hamid, K. Shahul; and Vijayan, B. "Antifertility Effect of *Andrographis paniculata* in Male Albino Rat." *Indian Journal of Experimental Biology* 28:421–26, May 1990.

Bieira, Paulo C.; Kubo, Isao; Kujime, Hiroshi; Yamagiwa, Yoshiro; and Kamikawa, Tadao. "Molluscicidal Acridone Alkaloids from *Angostura paniculata:* Isolation, Structures, and Synthesis." *Jounal of Natural Products* 55:1112–17, August 1992.

Choudhury, B. Roy, and Poddar, M. K. "Andrographolide and Kalmegh (*Andrographis paniculata*) Extract: *In Vivo* and *In Vitro* Effect on Hepatic Lipid Peroxidation." *Methods and Findings Experimental Clinical Pharmacology* 6:481–85, 1984.

Churvedi, G. N.; Tomar, G. S.; Tiwari, S. K.; and Singh, K. P. "Clinical Studies on Kalmegh (*Andrographis Paniculata* Nees) in Infective Hepatitis." *Ancient Science of Life: Journal of International Institute of Ayurveda* 2:208–11, 1983.

Gupta, Shashi; Choudhry, Mashkoor Ahmad; and Yadava, J. N. S. "Antidiarrhoeal Activity of Diterpenes of *Andrographis paniculata* (Kal-Megh) against *Escherichia coli* Enterotoxin in *in vivo* Models." *International Journal of Crude Drug Research* 28:273–83, 1990.

Madav, S.; Tripathi, H. C.; Mishra, Tandan; and Mishra, S. K. "Analgesic, Antipyretic, and Antiulcerogenic Effects of Andrographolide." *Indian Journal of Pharmacological Science* 57:121–125, 1995.

Matsuda, Takakuni; Kuroyanagi, Masanori; Sugiyama, Satoko; Umehara, Kaoru; Ueno, Akira; and Nishi, Kozaburo. "Cell Differentiation-Inducing Diterpenes from *Andrographis paniculata* Nees." *Chem Pharm Bulletin* 42:1216–25, 1994.

Puri, Anju; Saxena, Ragini; Saxena, R. P.; and Saxena, K. C. "Immunostimulant Agents From *Andrographis paniculata*." *Journal of Natural Products* 56:995–99, July 1993.

Sandberg, Finn. M.D. "Andrographidis herba Chuanxinlian." Austin, Texas: American Botanical Council.

Sharma, Anupam; Lal, Krishan and Handa, Sukhdev S. "Standardization of the

Indian Crude Drug Kalmegh by High Pressure Liquid Chromatographic Determination of Andrographolide." *Phytochemical Analysis* 3:129–31, 1992.

Shukla, Binduja; Visen, P. K. S.; Patnaik, G. K.; and Dhawan, B. N. "Choleratic Effect of Andrographolide in Rats and Guinea Pigs." *Planta Medica* 146–49, 1992.

Siripong, P.; Kongkathi, B.: Preechanukool, K.; Picha, P.; Tunsuwan, K.; and Taylor, W. C. "Cytotoxic Diterpenoid Constituents From *Andrographis paniculata* Nees Leaves." *Journal of the Scientific Society of Thailand* 18:187–94, 1992.

Zhao, Hua-yue, and Wei-yi, Fang. "Antithrombotic Effects of *Andrographis paniculata* Nees in Preventing Myocardial Infarction." *Chinese Medical Journal* 104:770–75, 1991.

_____. "Protective Effects of *Andrographis paniculata* Nees on Postinfarction Myocardium in Experimental Dogs." *Journal of Tongji Medical University* 10:212–17, 1990.

Biotechnology

Elkington, John. *The Gene Factory: Inside the Genetic and Biotechnololgy Business Revolution.* New York: Carroll and Graf Publishers, 1985.

Flam, Faye. "Chemical Prospectors Scour the Seas for Promising Drugs." *Science,* November 25, 1994, pp. 1324–25.

Hemmings, Brian A. "Akt Signaling: Linking Membrane Events to Life and Death Decisions." *Science,* January 31, 1997, pp. 628–30.

Huang, Xianming; Molema, Grietje; King, Steven; Watkins, Linda; Edington, Thomas S.; and Thorpe, Philip E. "Tumor Infarction in Mice by Antibody-Directed Targeting of Tissue Factor to Tumor Vasculature." *Science,* January 24, 1997, pp. 547–50.

"Infertility Is Linked to a Low-Calorie Diet." *Medical Herald,* February 1997, p. 48.

Jang, Meishiang; Cai, Lining; Udeani, George O.; Slowing, Karla V.; Thomas, Cathy F.; Beecher, Christopher W. W.; Fond, Harry H. S.; Farnsworth, Norman R.; Kinghorn, A. Douglas; Mehta, Rajendra G.; Moon, Richard C.; and John M. Pezzuto. "Cancer Chemopreventive Activity of Resveratrol, a Natural Product Derived From Grapes." *Science,* January 10, 1997, p. 218+.

Kabak, Joanne. "Menopause, Naturally: Some Things That Can Ease the Passage." *Newsday,* July 14, 1997, p. B13+.

Kapil, Aruna; Koul, I. B.; Banerjee, S. K.; and Gupta, B. D. "Antihepatotoxic Effects of Major Diterpenoid Constituents of *Andrographis paniculata.*" *Biochemical Pharmacology* 46:182–85, 1993.

Kenney, Martin. *Biotechnology: The University-Industrial Complex.* New Haven, Conn: Yale University Press, 1986.

Kerr, Kathleen. "Triple Threat to AIDS Touted." *Newsday,* June 20, 1997, p. A7.

_____. "FDA Issues HIV-Drugs Warning: Diabetes, Hypertension Side Effects of Protease Inhibitors." *Newsday*, June 12, 1997, p. A21.

Koutlas, Theodore C., ed. *The Mont Reid Surgical Handbook*. 3rd ed. St. Louis: Mosby, 1994.

Long, Irving. "Prostate Testing Touted." *Newsday*, May 28, 1997, p. A27.

Ma, Xinfang, and Babish, John G. "Activation of Signal Transduction Pathways by Dioxins." In *Molecular Biology Approaches to Toxicology*, A. Puga and K. B. Wallce, ed. Washington D.C.: Taylor and Francis, 1997.

Ma, Xinfang; Stoffregen, Dana A.; Wheelock, Geoffrey D.; Rininger, Joseph A.; and Babish, John G. "Discordant Hepatic Expression of the Cell Division Control Enzyme p34[cdc2] Kinase, Proliferating Cell Nuclear Antigen, p53 Tumor Suppressor Protein, and p21[Waf1] Cyclin-Dependent Kinase Inhibitory Protein After WY14,643 ([4-chloro-6-(2,3-xylidino)-2-pyrimidinylthio]acetic acid) Dosing to Rats." *Molecular Pharmacology*, 51:69–78, 1997.

Ma, Xingang; Mufti, Naheed A.; and Babish, John G. "Protein Tyrosine-Phosphorylation As an Indicator of 2,3,7,8-tetrachloro-p-dioxin Exposure *in vivo* and *in vitro*." *Biochemical and Biophysical Research Communications* 189:59–65, 1992.

Maccabe, Tom. "The Checkered Past of Children's Health." *Medical Herald*, June 1997, p. S-11.

Mangel, Charles, and Weisse, Allen B., M.D. *Medicine: The State of the Art*. New York: The Dial Press, 1984.

Marshall, Eliot. "Varmus to Rule in Fight Over Cell-Sorting Technology." *Science*, June 6, 1997, p. 1488+.

McAuliffe, Sharon, and McAuliffe, Kathleen. *Life for Sale*. New York: Coward, McCann and Geoghegan, 1981.

Nichols, Eve K. *Human Gene Therapy*. Cambridge, Mass.: Harvard University Press, 1988.

Rawls, Rebecca. "Optimistic About Antisense." *Chemical and Engineering News*, June 2, 1997, pp. 35–39.

Sharma, Anupam; Lal, Krishan; and Handa, Sukhdev S. "Standardization of the Indian Crude Drug Kalmegh by High Pressure Liquid Chromatographic Determiniation of Andrographolide." *Phytochemical Analysis* 3:129–31, 1992.

"Signal Transduction Research Brings Alum to Cold Spring Harbor." *Images*, Spring/Summer 1997, pp. 22–23.

Cancer

Cooke, Robert. "Enzyme May Hold Key to Breast Cancer." *Newsday*, April 2, 1997, p. A30.

Dermer, Dr. Gerald B. *The Immortal Cell: Why Cancer Research Fails*. Garden City Park, N.Y.: Avery Publishing Group, 1994.

Katzenstein, Larry. "Unraveling Cancer's Riddles." *American Health*, November 1994, p. 76.

Lane, William I., Ph.D. and Comac, Linda. *Sharks Don't Get Cancer.* Garden City Park, N.Y.: Avery Publishing Group, 1992.

——————. *Sharks Still Don't Get Cancer.* Garden City Park, N.Y.: Avery Publishing Group, 1996.

Morin, Patrice J.; Sparks, Andrew B.; Korinek, Vladimir; Barker, Mick; Clevers, Hans; Vogelstein, Bert; and Kinzler, Kenneth W. "Activation of β-Catenin-Tcf Signaling in Colon Cancer by Mutations in β-Catenin or APC." *Science*, March 21, 1997, pp. 1787–89.

Rininger, Joseph A.; Ma, Xinfang; Stoffregen, Dana A.; Wheelock, Geoffrey D.; and Babish, John G. "Chemical Carcinogenesis As a Consequence of Cell Cycle Dysregulation." In Proceedings of First World Molecular Toxicology Symposium, Sophia-Antipolis, France, 1997.

Rouhi, Maureen. "Change of Tactics in Cancer War Urged." *Chemical and Engineering News*, June 2, 1997, pp. 6–7.

Simone, Charles B., M.D. *Breast Health.* Garden City Park, N.Y.: Avery Publishing Group, 1995.

Steele, Glen D. Jr., M.D.; Jessup, L. Milburn M.D.; Winchester, David P., M.D.; Murphy, Gerald P. M.D.; and Menck, Herman R., M.B.A. *Clinical Highlights From the National Cancer Data Base: 1995.* Atlanta: American Cancer Society/American College of Surgeons Commission on Cancer, 1995.

Chinese Medicine

East Asian Medical Studies Society. *Fundamentals of Chinese Medicine.* Brookline, Mass.: Paradigm Publications, 1985.

Maciocia, Giovanni. *The Practice of Chinese Medicine: The Treatment of Diseases With Acupuncture and Chinese Herbs.* Edinburgh, Scotland: Churchill Livingstone, 1994.

Teeguarden, Ron. *Chinese Tonic Herbs.* Japan Publications, 1984.

Willard, Terry. *Textbook of Advanced Herbology.* Calgary, Alberta: Wild Rose College of Natural Healing, 1992.

Heart Disease and Strokes

Cohen, Paula. "A Promising Treatment for Strokes." *Newsday*, February 22, 1997, p. B11.

Hademenos, George J. "The Biophysics of Stroke." *American Scientist*, May/June 1997, 226–35.

"Health Watch: Bypass Surgery Aid." *Newsday*, September 16, 1997, p. C9.

"Heart-Attack Drugs Help Those With Lung Clots." *Newsday*, August 5, 1997, p. A15.

"Heart Ills World's Top Death Cause." *Newsday*, May 3, 1997, p. A8.

Samiei, Mitra; Daya-Makin, Maleki; Clark-Lewis, Ian; and Pelech, Steven L. "Platelet-Activating Factor and Thrombin-Induced Stimulation of p34[cdc2]-Cyclin Histone H1 Kinase Activity in Platelets." *The Journal of Biological Chemistry* 266:14889–92, 1991.

"Study Gives Edge to Angioplasty." *Newsday*, June 5, 1997, p. A17.

Talan, Jamie, and Vincent, Stuart. "Popular Diet Pills Recalled." *Newsday*, September 16, 1997, p. A5+.

Wang, Dao-wen, and Zhao, Hua-yue. "Experimental Studies on Prevention of Atherosclerotic Arterial Stenosis and Restenosis After Angioplasty With *Andrographis paniculata* Nees and Fish Oil." In *Journal of Tongji Medical University* 13:193–98, 1993.

Wertenbaker, Lael. *To Mend the Heart: The Dramatic Story of Cardiac Surgery and Its Pioneers*. New York: Viking Press, 1980.

Herbal Medicine

Agosta, William. *Bombardier Beetles and Fever Trees: A Close-Up Look at Chemical Warfare and Signals in Animals and Plants*. New York: Addison-Wesley Publishing Company, 1996.

Antol, Marie Nadine. *Healing Teas: How to Prepare and Use Teas to Maximize Your Health*. Garden City Park, N.Y.: Avery Publishing Group, 1996.

Blum, Murray. "Nature's Chemical Arsenal." *Chemical and Engineering News*, July 1, 1996, pp. 32+.

Bricklin, Mark. *The Practical Encyclopedia of Natural Healing*. Emmaus, Penn.: Rodale Press, 1976.

Castleman, Michael. "Consumer Savy: Claim Check." *Prevention's Guide to Natural Healing Breakthroughs*, September 1997, pp. 20–23.

Echeverri, Ana P., M.D. "Phyto-Est for Menopausal Relief." *Nutriceutical News International*, vol. 1, Nos. 3 and 4, pp. 4–5.

Elias, Jason, and Masline, Shelagh Ryan. *The A to Z Guide to Healing Herbal Remedies*. New York: Dell Publishing, 1995.

Foster, Steven. "Echinacea: The Cold and Flu Remedy." *Alternative and Complementary Therapies*, June/July 1995, p. 254–57.

Griggs, Barbara. *Green Pharmacy: The History and Evolution of Western Herbal Medicine*. Rochester, Vt.: Healing Arts Press, 1991.

Huang, Kee Chang, M.D. *The Pharmacology of Chinese Herbs*. Boca Raton, Fla.: CRC Press, 1993.

Joyce, Christopher. *Earthly Goods: Medicine Hunting in the Rainforest*. New York: Little Brown, 1994.

McGuffin, Michael, ed. *American Herbal Products Association's Botanical Safety Handbook*. Boca Raton, Fla., CRC Press, 1997.

Mervis, Jeffrey. "Ancient Remedy Performs New Tricks." *Science,* August 2, 1996.

Mindell, Earl, R. Ph.D. *Earl Mindell's Herb Bible.* New York: Simon and Schuster, 1992.

"Old Chinese Herbal Medicine Used for Fever Yields Possible New Alzheimer Disease Therapy." *Journal of the American Medical Association,* March 12, 1997, p. 776.

Rao, Linda. "An Aisle-land Adventure." *Prevention's Guide to Natural Healing Breakthroughs,* September 1997, pp. 26–37.

Reid, Daniel. *A Handbook of Chinese Healing Herbs.* Boston, Mass. Shambhala Press, 1995.

Rouhi, A. Maureen. "Seeking Drugs in Natural Products." *Chemical and Engineering News,* April 7, 1997, pp. 14 + .

Squires, Sally. "The New Medicine." *Modern Maturity,* September/October 1996, p. 69.

Sutarjadi, M. H.; Bendryman, Santosa; and Dyatmiko, W. "Immunomodulatory Activity of *Piper betle, Zingiber aromatica, Andrographis paniculata, Allium sativum,* and *Oldenlandia corymbosa* Grown in Indonesia." In *Planta Medica,* supplement issue 2, 1991.

Teeguarden, Ron. *Chinese Tonic Herbs.* Japan Publications, 1984.

Unger, Michael. "LI Herbal Remedies a Budding Business." *Newsday,* August 4, 1997, p. C6.

Vedavathy, S., and Rao, K. N. "Antipyretic Activity of Six Indigenous Medicinal Plants of Tirumala Hills, Andhra Pradesh, India." *Journal of Ethnopharmacology* 33 (1991), pp. 193–96.

Waxman, Sharon. "The Healing Power of Herbs." *Good Housekeeping,* November 1996, p. 104 + .

Wicht, Max. *Herbal Drugs and Phytopharmaceuticals.* Boca Raton, Fla.: CRC Press, 1995.

Willard, Terry. *Textbook of Advanced Herbology.* Calgary, Alberta: Wild Rose College of Natural Healing, 1992.

Miscellaneous

Bagla, Pallava. "Malaria Fighters Gather at Site of Early Victory." *Science,* September 5, 1977, p. 1437.

Brookes, Vincent J., and Jacobs, Morris B. *Poisons: Properties, Chemical Identification, Symptoms, and Emergency Treatment.* Princeton, N.J.: D. Van Nostrand Company, 1958.

———. "Can Stopping Gene Expression From Changing Keep the Blood Flowing?" *Images,* Spring/Summer 1997, pp. 2–5.

Cimons, Marlene. "Can an Experimental Drug Help You?" *Good Housekeeping,* April 1997, pp. 153–54.

Clements, Mark, and Hales, Dianne. "How Healthy Are We?" *Parade*, September 7, 1997, pp. 4–7.

Cohen, Jon. "Exclusive License Rankles Genome Researchers." *Science*, June 6, 1997, p. 1469.

Cooke, Robert. "Key in TB Fight." *Newsday*, June 10, 1997, p. A6.

_____. "Fighting Drug-Resistant Disease." *Newsday*, August 5, 1997, p. A3.

Holt, Stephen, M.D. *Soya for Health: The Definitive Medical Guide.* Larchmont, N.Y.: Mary Ann Liebert, 1996.

Lin, Wendy. "Life After the Diet Drugs." *Newsday*, September 22, 1997, pp. B13 +.

Myers, Allen R., M.D. *Medicine.* Philadelphia: Harwal Publishing, 1994.

"New Terpene Blocks Protein Phosphatase." *Chemical and Engineering News*, September 16, 1996, p. 28.

Ochs, Ridgely. "Antibiotic-Resistant Strep Found." *Newsday*, September 11, 1997, p. A21.

Preston, Richard. *The Hot Zone.* New York: Doubleday, 1994.

Reno, Robert. "Drug Companies Playing Pusher on the Airwaves." *Newsday*, August 14, 1997, p. A59.

Ricks, Delthia. "Drug Said to Attack Arthritis Rather Than Just Symptoms." *Newsday*, July 17, 1997, p. A20.

Rininger, J. A.; Goldsworthy, T. L.; and Babish, J. G. "Time Course Comparison of Cell-Cycle Protein Expression Following Partial Hepatectomy and WY14,643-induced Hepatic Cell Proliferation in F344 Rats." *Carcinogenesis* 18, 1997.

Rininger, Joseph A.; Wheelock, Geoffrey D.; Ma, Xinfang; and Babish, John G. "Discordant Expressing of the Cyclin-Dependent Kinases and Cyclins in Rat Liver Following Acute Administration of the Hepatocarcinogen [4-chloro-6-(2,3-xylidino) -2-pyrimidinylthio] acetic acid Dosing to Rats." *Biochemical Pharmacology* 52:1749–55, 1996.

Rondberg, Terry A., D.C. *Chiropractic First. Chiropractic Journal*, 1996.

Sabiston, David C. Jr., M.D., and Lyerly, H. Kim, M.D., eds. *Textbook of Surgery: Pocket Companion.* W. B. Saunders Company, Philadelphia: 1992.

Sedgwick, John. "Junk Medicine." *Self*, August 1997, pp. 145 +.

Singer, Charles. *A History of Biology.* New York: Abelard-Schuman, 1962.

Stix, Gary. "Profile: Wayne B. Jonas." *Scientific American*, October 1996, p. 52 +.

Ubell, Earl. "What Vitamins Can Do for You." *Parade*, October 13, 1996, pp. 12–13.

Western Medicine

Bedeschi, Giulio. *Science of Medicine.* New York: Franklin Watts, 1975.

Cohen, Daniel. *The Last Hundred Years: Medicine.* New York: M. Evans and Company, 1981.

"Doctors Rap Managed Care Shortcomings." *The Medical Herald*, June 1997; p. 32.

Drake, Donald, and Uhlman, Marian. *Making Medicine, Making Money.* Kansas City, Mo.: Andrews and McMeel, 1993.

Gordon, Benjamin Lee, M.D., F.I.C.S. *Medieval and Renaissance Medicine.* New York: Philosophical Library, 1959.

Tapley, Donald, E., M.D. *Columbia University College of Physicians and Surgeons Complete Home Medical Guide.* New York: Crown Publishers, 1995.

Appendix A:
Technical Data

Peppermint Oil's Mechanism of Action

Peppermint oil contains menthol, which is a cyclical monoterpene that, when taken orally, is rapidly absorbed from the upper portions of the small intestine. The cyclical monoterpene content of essential oils is believed to exert pharmacologic effects, including the modulation of gastrointestinal smooth muscle function.

Toxicological Studies of *Andrographis paniculata*

Formal toxicological studies in animal models and in animal and human clinical trials confirmed that andrographolide has very low toxicity. Rats and rabbits administered 1 gram per kilogram of body weight (g/kg) of an *Andrographis paniculata* extract once a day for seven days showed no adverse effects. Body weights were not affected and blood counts were normal, as were hepatic and renal functions and the histology of important organs. Furthermore, at these levels the animals remained energetic. Very large doses of 10 g/kg given to mice did entail some decreased motor activity and lethargy, but none of the animals died and there was no damage to major organs. Some toxicity did become apparent with huge doses of andrographolides; at 13.4 g/kg, 50 percent of the tested animals died.

Once safety had been established, scientists began to look at the pharmacokinetics and biodisposition of andrographolide in various organs of the body. Experiments using radiolabeled andrographolide revealed that after intravenous injection, the compound becomes widely distributed. It penetrates the blood-brain barrier rather quickly and concentrates in the central nervous system — particularly the spinal cord. High concentrations are also seen in the colon, spleen, heart, lungs, and kidneys. Six hours after injection, the highest concentrations of andrographolide sulfate were found in the rectum and duodenum.

Andrographolide is absorbed and excreted from the body fairly rapidly: 80 percent of the dose is removed from the body within eight hours via the urine and gastrointestinal tract, with excretion rates of more than 90 percent of the compound within forty-eight hours.

Clinical Tests of *Andrographis paniculata*'s Antifertility Effects

When high doses of *Andrographis paniculata* were administered to animals, both antifertility and pregnancy-terminating effects were seen. Spermatogenesis ceased when dry leaf powder was fed to male albino rats for sixty days. Investigators noted degenerative changes in organs and tissues related to sperm production. In female mice, injection of a large dose of *Andrographis paniculata* decoction prevented implantation of the fertilized egg and caused abortion at every gestational period.

Tests of *Andrographis paniculata*'s Antipyretic Ability

In one test, plant materials were dried and powdered and an extract was prepared and filtered. Fever was induced in rats by injecting brewer's yeast subcutaneously into the animals' backs. The animals showed a mean increase in temperature of 1.45° C. after injections of Brewer's yeast. Rats whose temperatures had increased 1.2° C. or more twenty hours after the injections received *Andrographis paniculata* extracts. A control group received equal amounts of the extract vehicle. Administration of andrographolide at doses of 100 and 300 mg/kg significantly lowered fever. At oral doses of 300 mg/kg, fever-lowering was comparable to the effect of aspirin. Furthermore, in studies evaluating small animals' reaction time to certain physical stimuli, extracts were found to have analgesic activity. In addition, the extracts did not appear toxic; they were well tolerated at oral doses up to 600 mg/kg.

Tests of *Andrographis paniculata*'s Immune-Stimulating Activity

Research was conducted by the Center for Research and Development of Traditional Medicines, Alrlangga University, Indonesia, and reported in

Planta Medica. Using mice, the researchers studied the immunomodulatory activities of certain plants, including *Andrographis paniculata.* The investigators found that the water nonsoluble fraction stimulated phagocytosis. The nonsoluble fraction also stimulated cellular immune suppression, but the water soluble fraction was found to cause cellular immune suppression alone.

In one study, 50 gm of the herb was boiled in 1,000 ml of water and then strained. The resulting decoction was shown to increase leukocytes' ability to engulf *Staphylococcus aureus.* When humans took the decoction orally, the skin reaction to tuberculotoxin was boosted. It has also been reported that extracts of the herb enhance cell-mediated immunity, as measured by cutaneous responses to tuberculin toxins.

In addition, studies in mice showed that andrographolides increased the serum level of an enzyme that destroys the cell walls of certain bacteria. When sulphonated andrographolide was administered to rabbits or mice continually, certain immune system cells' ability to fight *Pneumococcus* or *Staphylococcus aureus* improved. It appears that andrographis is a mighty, versatile booster of immune functions.

Andrographis Paniculata As a Hepatoprotective Agent

Usually, carbon tetrachloride will inhibit hepatic protein synthesis and cause a disturbance in hepatic electrolyte balance. Dosing with andrographis extracts for seven days elevated cellular antioxidant defenses and reduced the peroxidation that results from a toxic dose of carbon tetrachloride. Peroxidation is associated with oxidative changes in the body — changes that generally cause disease states, are responsible for aging, and contribute to vascular disease.

Investigators at the University of Calcutta studied the effects of *Andrographis paniculata* leaf extract and pure andrographolide on carbon-tetrachloride-induced lipid peroxidation in vivo and in vitro. In vitro, lipid peroxidation was completely normalized by the leaf extract and the pure andrographolide. When the concentration of carbon tetrachloride was high, peroxidation was significantly increased in the presence of andrographolide but not in the presence of the leaf extract. Apparently, the leaves of *Andrographis paniculata* afford more protection against carbon tetrachloride toxicity than does the bitter principle alone.

In in vivo studies with rats, it became obvious that carbon tetrachloride increases lipid peroxidation, while *Andrographis paniculata* leaf extract and andrographolide decrease the peroxidation in a concentration-dependent manner. When the leaf extract has been administered, carbon tetrachloride does not produce appreciable changes in lipid peroxidation at any concentration. Because carbon tetrachloride initiates action very rapidly, neither *Andrographis paniculata* leaf extract nor andrographolide protect against lipid peroxidation when either is administered at the same time as the carbon tetrachloride. Long-term administration of either substance prior to exposure does not prevent carbon-tetrachloride-induced lipid peroxidation. When rats were pretreated for fifteen consecutive days and then exposed to carbon tetrachloride, lipid peroxidation was unchanged. If the carbon tetrachloride is administered immediately after the last treatment with either leaf extract or andrographolide, lipid peroxidation increases tremendously — 50 or 37 percent, respectively.

Tests of *Andrographis paniculata*'s Effectiveness in Infective Hepatitis

In one study, acute hepatitis was chemically induced in rats, and hepatoprotective activity was monitored by examining blood samples and abnormal changes in the rats' liver cells. Treatment with 400 mg/kg intraperitoneally or 800 mg/kg orally before administration of the chemical hepatitis-inducer led to normalization of the toxin-induced increase in all biochemical parameters. It also significantly reduced the toxin-induced abnormalities in cells.

Understanding Liver Cancer

Studies of a certain dioxin's relationship to hepatic intracellular signal transduction pathways were reported in a toxicology textbook in 1997. The dioxin's effect on signaling pathways and cell cycle control enzymes provides an explanation for the variety of biological effects observed with exposure.

In recent studies of substances carcinogenic to the liver, researchers demonstrated that, among other effects, the carcinogen produced increases in CDK-1. CDK-1 or its activity has been reported to be elevated in cancer cells and after acute and subchronic exposure to TCDD, a dioxin (a very toxic chemical that can cause cancer). The stimulation of two CDKs by TCDD is consistent with a mechanism of action of TCDD toxicity associated with the stimulation of cellular proliferation.

Evidence for Green Tea's Anticancer Effects

S. Okabe, M.D., and his colleagues have shown that green tea can inhibit the growth of a human lung cancer cell line (type PC9). The inhibitory effect has been identified as involving G 2/M arrest in the cell cycle. Although EGCg has been shown to inhibit neoplastic growth in the skin, stomach, duodenum, colon, liver, lung and pancreas of animals, it did not appear to be effective in inhibiting the growth of lymphoma, spontaneous mammary cancer, or bladder cancer. EGCg can, however, inhibit the metastasis of melanoma B16 cells to the lung.

Andrographolide for Indigestion

Researchers note that consumption of alui would not provide andrographolide in amounts as large as those used in this test. They suggest that the combined effect of the andrographolide analogs may be greater than any single analog.

Andrographis paniculata and Cobra Venom

Because the herb has distinct antithrombolytic activity in several animal models, it has been suggested that injections of the extract may inhibit the pulmonary thromboembolisms formed as a result of thrombinlike enzymes in snake venom.

The Role of p53 in the Cell Cycle

P53 functions as a genomic guardian, preventing cell cycle progression in the event of DNA damage. In vitro, both p53 and Rb proteins have been shown to arrest cells in the G_1 and G_2 phases of the cell cycle to prevent unscheduled cellular proliferation.

Using signal transduction technology, scientists found that the molecule fundamental to coordination of events involved in cell division is p34; it activates the p53 molecule to halt cell replication. Abnormal p34 levels have been found in approximately 90 percent of breast tumor cells.

In 1995, the use of p34 as an early diagnostic or prognostic marker for cancer was granted foreign patent protection. The International Preliminary Examining Authority deemed the p34 protein "novel, inventive, and patentable."

Enzymes in the Signaling Process

Enzymes called CDKs, along with the cyclin and CDK inhibitory proteins, control and coordinate the molecular events in the cell cycle. Timely passage from the G_1 phase into the DNA synthesis phase, execution of mitosis, and creation of a daughter cell are all dependant upon CDK activity. The expression and regulation of this activity is of utmost importance in guarding integrity of the genome, the complete set of chromosomes with its associated genes.

Information About Herbal Doses

Manipulation of herbal doses may play a role in the response to therapy. The concepts behind acute, subacute, and chronic dosing schedules with herbs remain empiric and are worthy of further detailed study. Treatment with herbals that have variable dose response and variable efficacy can assist in defining safe and effective interventions that have the possibility of revolutionizing cancer therapy.

New Information About TCDD Toxicity

TCDD toxicities are believed to be receptor mediated. Researchers are tempted to infer that the stimulus for increased expression of CDK-1 provided by TCDD is initiated by the interaction of receptors specific for materials foreign to living organisms. This interaction provides the cell with a continuous proliferative signal that mimics the aberrant signaling pathways in transformed cells.

Understanding Hemostasis

One of the factors that contributes to hemostasis is the formation of a fibrin clot. Fibrin is a protein that forms a fibrous network in the coagulation of blood. The process of coagulation involves the conversion of inactive substances to their active state through the action of enzymes.

When, for instance, platelets are activated, they link and position the clot where it is needed.

Free-floating or unnecessary fibrin would result in clots that obstruct the flow of blood. The primary mechanism for inhibiting fibrin is dissolution by plasmin. This substance circulates in its inactive form — plasminogen, which is found within each fibrin clot. Proper levels are maintained through feedback loops and crossover effects involving both amplification and inhibition.

Tissue plasminogen activator (TPA) is sometimes used to treat people in the early stages of a heart attack or stroke. Its use can, however, lead to dangerous bleeding within the brain. This intracerebral hemorrhage can lead to a stroke. Nevertheless, in June 1996, the FDA approved TPA to treat ischemic strokes. In these cases, which account for 80 percent of strokes, brain tissue dies because the blood supply is cut off by a clot or a narrowed blood vessel. In order for treatment to be effective, TPA must be administered within three hours of the onset of stroke. TPA should not be used by people who have suffered a ruptured vessel in the brain.

Experiments Demonstrating *Andrographis paniculata*'s Ability to Prevent Platelet Aggregation

One test of *Andrographis paniculata* was conducted on sixteen dogs: There were eight dogs in a control group and eight in the test group. The test group received 1 ml injections containing 1 g of a water-soluble component of the root of *Andrographis paniculata*. The crude extract was found to inhibit aggregation and adhesion of platelets. The extract also activated the breakdown of fibrin, thus reducing the possibility of clotting.

In both in vivo and in vitro studies, investigators have observed that extracts of *Andrographis paniculata* can inhibit certain forms of platelet aggregation. The investigators also examined the herb's effect on fibrinolysis. During this process, fibrin is broken into soluble substances by an enzyme. Investigators reported a 32 percent decrease in euglobulin lysis time, a measure of fibrinolysis. Euglobulins are precipitated by diluting and acidifying the plasma. The euglobulin fraction is relatively free of fibrinolysis inhibitors. The fraction is clotted with thrombin, and the time it takes for that clot to dissolve is measured. A shortened time indicates increased activity of the enzyme that breaks down fibrin. Results of the experiment indicate that extracts of *Andrographis paniculata* can facilitate the breakdown of clots. The researchers concluded that the herb might be beneficial in preventing and treating arterial thrombotic diseases.

Eight human volunteers and sixty-one blood samples were investigated to observe the effect of the dietary supplement *Andrographis paniculata* on platelet function in vitro and in vivo. Studies revealed that the crude extract could significantly inhibit certain forms of platelet aggregation. The potency of the extract seemed somewhat stronger than in vitro injections of two drugs commonly used to inhibit platelet aggregation, but the difference was not statistically significant. A dose-dependent effect was demonstrated; the effect was rapid, indicating quick absorption, but this was short-lived: Twelve hours after withdrawing the herbal extract, the one-minute and five-minute aggregation rates increased by 18.67 percent and 36.63 percent, respectively, compared to the lowest aggregation rate after administration.

In another study, sixty-three patients with cardiac and cerebral vascular disease received 5 mg of the herbal extract per kilogram of body weight three times a day. Within three hours, a 15 percent inhibition of platelet aggregation time was observed. Thirty-three of the patients were observed for seven days. At the end of the week, platelet accumulation time had decreased to 64 percent of the mean predose level. None of the patients displayed any adverse side effects. Investigators observed that *Andrographis paniculata* inhibited the platelets' release of substances that initiate blood clotting. These effects were observed by studying canals that exist in platelets, which are the origin of these aggretory compounds.

The Role of *Andrographis paniculata* in Myocardial Infarction

In one study, dogs with myocardial infarction received intravenous injections of a watery extract of *Andrographis paniculata*. In the treated group favorable changes in hormonelike substances called prostaglandins occurred and platelet clumping was interfered with through the administration of andrographis. These changes resulted in a reduction in the size of the area of decreased blood supply.

When the coronary arteries are obstructed by clots or coronary spasm, an electrocardiagram (ECG) shows S-T segment elevation. The elevation of the S-T segment in the treated animals was lower than in the andrographis-treated control group. On an ECG, Q waves appear where the S-T segments fall; the Q wave appeared in only one dog. The myocardial structure surrounding the initially appearing ischemic area (the reversibly damaged area) became relatively normal. The degree of myocardial degeneration and necrosis in the central part of the ischemic area was mild. These data suggest that in cases of myocardial infarction, *Andrographis paniculata* may limit the expansion of ischemia, exert marked protective effect on ischemic heart muscle, and demonstrate a weak fibrinolytic, or blood-thinning, action.

Testing the Role of *Andrographis paniculata* in Fighting HIV

In December 1995, researchers at the National Institutes of Health reported that certain immune or T cells infected with HIV-1 accumulate high levels of hyperphosphorylated CDK-1 and cyclin B. The research revealed that the AIDS virus's ability to kill cells is strongly linked to the continued over-expression of CDK-1 and cyclin B in the infected immune cell. Agents that can block phosphorylation attenuate the disease state. Such agents belong to a new class of antiviral compounds called tyrosine kinase inhibitors, which includes andrographolides. In April 1992, NIH researchers reported that these inhibitors can halt the disease-causing elements associated with HIV-1. Basically, these compounds are amino acids that inhibit enzymes involved in the production of high-energy phosphates.

Early observations have been made of the first antiviral agent to demonstrate that tyrosine kinase inhibition is indeed a mechanism for combating HIV infection. An extract of the herb *Andrographis paniculata* appears to achieve this effect. The herb seems to be specific for HIV-1 infected cells because of its ability to inhibit CDK-1. Present in insignificant amounts in normal cells, CDK-1's concentration and activity are dramatic in cells infected with the AIDS virus.

An herbal extract of andrographis was found to decrease the expression of both CDK-1 and cyclin B. In addition, cooperative research at the National Cancer Institute has shown that androgapholide inhibits HIV's toxic effect on cells by inhibiting an enzyme called c-mos. C-mos is involved in HIV-1 propagation and T-cell death. Normally found only in cells in the reproductive system, c-mos is not expressed in CD4 + cells or other body cells. When CD4 cells are infected by the HIV-1 virus, c-mos expression is activated.

According to Dr. David I. Cohen of NIH's Laboratory of Tumor Biology, "...expression of c-mos is tightly linked to the ability of the virus to replicate in T cells and to kill them. Since an ideal cellular target for drug therapy would be one that is not essential for normal cellular growth but required for HIV-1 cell killing and viral replication, we believe that we have identified such a target in c-mos kinase." Because andrographolide seems to inhibit this enzyme, it can support normal immune function. An extract of *Andrographis paniculata* has already demonstrated activity against c-mos kinase and has been shown to inhibit HIV-1 propagation in laboratory studies. "We envision that the inhibition of c-mos kinase may drastically limit the ability of HIV-1 virus to replicate in the infected individual and also further inhibit replicating virus from killing CD4+ and T cells," said Dr. Cohen.

A Hypothesis for *Andrographis paniculata*'s Mechanism of Action in AIDS

The herbal extract appears to induce apoptosis, or programmed cell death, in cells infected with HIV. Researchers hypothesize that apoptotic signals generated by the virus may be transmitted to uninfected immune cells. This would explain the vast T-cell destruction caused by HIV infection, which is far out of proportion to the amount of virus present.

Boswellia

Boswellic acids and related compounds appear to be inhibitors of leukotriene production, and they directly inhibit the 5-lipoxygenase enzyme without affecting the activity of cyclooxygenase enzyme activities. This means that boswellic acids and associated compounds may be specific inhibitors of the inflammatory mediating leukotrienes, but they do not exert significant effects on prostaglandin synthesis.

Echinacea

Laboratory experiments indicate that echinacea may enhance T-cell function, enhance neutrophil function, and promote antibody binding.

Evening Primrose Oil

The focus of attention in evening primrose oil as a health-giving constituent is gamma-linolenic acid, which is a precursor of prostaglandin E1.

Fennel

Fennel oil has the ability to block calcium movement in ionic channels in cells and cause smooth muscle relaxation.

St. John's Wort

The active constituents of St. John's wort are believed to include flavonoids and xanthones. It is believed that these substances function as inhibitors of monoamine oxidase.

Appendix B:
DSHEA

"The Dietary Supplement and Health Education Act:
Far-Reaching Consequences for Consumers and Manufacturers"
by Stephen Holt, M.D.
Reprinted with permission from *Alternatives*,
Mary Ann Liebert, Inc., Publisher

The Dietary Supplement Health and Education Act of 1994 (DSHEA) could revolutionize the regulation of the use of dietary supplements. Consumers, health professionals, and manufacturers and distributors of such products are not sure about the content and implications of this legislation. While the Act provides new marketing opportunities for dietary supplements — and perhaps more informed use of such supplements by consumers — it is the first step in regulatory control of the rapidly expanding dietary supplement industry.

The past several decades have seen a growing awareness of the key role nutrition plays in the quality of our health; it is now widely recognized, for example, that low-fat diets can help prevent certain cancers and heart diseases. As manufacturers of health foods and nutritional supplements sought to bring this information to the attention of the public — including, in some cases, hyperbole about "brain food" and other questionable claims — Congress began to question whether health claims should be allowed for foods and supplements. Congress passed the Nutritional Labeling and Education Act (NLEA) in 1990 in an effort to provide the Food and Drug Administration (FDA) with the tools and direction it needed to determine which health claims could properly be made. The FDA took a position in response to the NLEA, which many, including some in Congress, took to reflect an overeagerness to place undue restrictions upon claims made for dietary supplements. In response to this concern, and buoyed by an unusually strong public response, Congress passed the Dietary Supplement Health and Education Act of 1994 (DSHEA).

The DSHEA sought to moderate the approach to the regulation of dietary supplements embodied in the FDA's proposed regulations under the NLEA. One of the key issues is the standard of proof a manufacturer needs to meet in order to make a health claim. The NLEA required a manufacturer to show "significant scientific agreement" supporting the proposed health claim. This standard was an effort to create an intermediate threshold for the approval of health claims on foods. Congress was concerned about radical and unregulated claims being made for some health foods, but it did not wish to place the expensive and technical requirements upon supplements that it had placed on drugs. The standard requiring "significant scientific agreement" was unsatisfactory to the health food industry and many consumers. One problem with the standard was that it was not one with a history developed at law, so that the meaning of the standard was unclear; it could be interpreted as a requirement as simple as a dozen published articles in agreement with the claim, or as difficult as agreement by a National Institutes of Health (NIH) consensus panel. The standard also raised concerns, given the hesitation and conservatism of the scientific community toward recognizing the positive health benefits of nutritional interventions, that this would create an unduly high threshold. The lobbying, which ultimately resulted in the passage of the DSHEA, arose in large measure because of dissatisfaction with this requirement.

Unfortunately, the supporters of the DSHEA were not able to revise this standard. The DSHEA thus took other approaches to moderate the severity of this standard. One approach taken was to allow a manufacturer of a supplement to make truthful structure and function claims — claims that do not describe an indication or make a specific "health" claim — without requiring that those claims be subjected to regulatory approval by the FDA. A manufacturer can claim, for example, that antioxidants help remove oxidized material in the body, but could not, without approval of a health claim, state that antioxidants have a beneficial effect in preventing cancer.

The DSHEA also allows manufacturers and distributors of supplements greater latitude in informing the public about the health benefits of their products. The law regulating claims made for food and drugs prescribes what can be placed on the label—the packaging affixed to the product—the separate materials that are distributed with the product, such as package inserts or sales brochures. As discussed below, the DSHEA removed many types of literature from the definition of labeling, allowing consumers greater access to materials describing the health benefits of supplements, and allowing other members of the industry to make claims for products which the manufacturers of the products could not.

The Findings Section

The findings section of the Act deserves special consideration because it reflects the underlying issues that Congress was addressing when the legislation was under consideration.

Several important issues emerged in the findings section of the DSHEA. There was a general recognition that dietary supplements have been shown to be of use in the prevention of chronic disease and an inference emerged that their use, in an appropriate manner, may reduce the prevalence of several common chronic disorders. The notion that this approach could lead to a reduction in long-term health care costs was entertained but nutrieconomic studies—investigations of the cost effectiveness of nutriceuticals—were not included in the Act.

The rights of consumers to make informed decisions about preventive health care strategies was revisited in the Act, with an emphasis on the importance of the quest for scientific knowledge about the benefits or hazards of dietary supplements. It was noted that approximately one half of all Americans may use dietary supplements to improve their nutrition and that much greater relevance is being placed on alternative health care providers because of the high cost of conventional medical interventions. This reinforced the need to protect a consumer's right to safe dietary supplements. These and other factors underscored the need for a framework to be established that supersedes what may perceived as "ad hoc" regulatory policies.

Defining a Dietary Supplement

The most important aspect of the characterization of a "dietary supplement" by the DSHEA is that the dietary supplement is *not* a new drug or a food additive. Section 3 of the Act refers to a dietary supplement as a substance intended to supplement the diet and that contains one or more of the following components or characteristics: vitamins, minerals, herbs, botanicals, amino acids. It also is a substance for use by humans that supplements the diet by increasing total dietary intake or it is a concentrate, metabolite, constituent, extract, or combination of any of the above mentioned ingredients.

Certain qualifications apply to this definition, including the necessity for labeling of a product as a dietary supplement and not representing the product as a conventional food or as a sole item of a meal or of the diet. Dietary supplements under this definition are to be supplied in dosage forms, such as capsules, tablets, liquids, gels, or powders.

Section 3(b) of the DSHEA clearly distinguishes between a dietary supplement and a food additive. Food additives are subject to strict regulation in a defined process of premarket approval by the FDA. This provision is very important to the health food industry and it prevents the FDA from claiming that certain dietary supplements are food additives that require a process of strict regulatory approval.

Safety of Dietary Supplements

The Secretary of Health and Human Services (HHS) may take action against a supplement which presents a significant or unreasonable risk of injury, or, in the case of a new dietary product, where there is inadequate documentation of safety. The Secretary may also suspend the sale of a dietary supplement if an imminent threat to public safety exists. If the FDA deems a product to be unsafe, then the burden of proof rests with the FDA to demonstrate any alleged lack of safety. The Act demands that the FDA both provide ten days notice to the manufacturer or distributor of a product that a civil proceeding is imminent and grant an opportunity to discuss such action.

The Act provides useful guidelines as to what constitutes an unsafe product. If a substance is considered to present a significant or unreasonable risk of illness or injury under the conditions of the recommended use on the label or in accompanying labeling, then it is deemed unsafe.

The FDA has to judge the safety of a product, in part, based on the labeling. This should encourage manufacturers to apply warning statements on products. This will lead to safer use of dietary supplements because warnings and cautions are quite permissible, and specific dosage instructions should be disclosed by manufacturers or distributors wherever possible.

The Act recognizes that public policy should be that a consumer could make an informed judgment about the use of a dietary supplement based on accurate information on the benefits of dietary supplements. This section is very important for those individuals in the industry who are involved in the creation of a platform for the advertising or promotion of dietary supplements and it presents many opportunities for creative marketing of dietary supplements. Such creativity should occur with conformity to the Act.

Dietary Supplements and Literature

Formerly, the use of literature by the distributors of dietary supplements that contained health claims was not allowed. Section 5 of the DSHEA has changed this situation radically. A publication that is reprinted in its entirety can be used in a retail environment providing certain specific guidelines are followed. The Act indicates that the literature can be an article, a publication, a book chapter, or an official abstract of a peer-reviewed scientific publication that was prepared by the author or the editors of the publications. This area of the legislation will be open to interpretation, and it will be a likely focus of further contention and definition.

The literature that can be provided to a consumer in a retail outlet must not be false or misleading. Retailers of dietary supplements have some responsibility to be cognizant of what is being sold in their outlets. This means that if a government agency was to determine that dietary supplement literature was false, there is a potential liability for the retailer. The literature must not promote a particular manufacturer or brand of dietary supplement. The Act indicates that the literature should be displayed or presented with other items on the same subject so as to present a "balanced view" of the available scientific information on the dietary supplement. This is a very difficult problem with "unique" products which may be proprietary formulations or combinations. There may be only one type of a dietary supplement for an author to discuss. If the literature used to sell dietary supplements is displayed in an establishment, such as a retail outlet, then the literature has to be physically separate from the dietary supplement.

It seems likely that the responsible production of an accurate product monograph for consumers would be perceived as appropriate, but no test cases exist under the new legislation where "expanded" literature use as labeling has been used. This portion of the Act does not prevent the sale of books or publications by purveyors of dietary supplements.

Section 5 of the Act is intimately related to dietary supplement claims and labeling. This area of the legislation provides an exemption from the former basic rule that information used to sell a dietary supplement is considered to be "labeling," when it is provided by a manufacturer, distributor, retailer, or even perhaps a health care professional. The Act does not enter into specific detail concerning situations where health care professionals may be selling their own brand of dietary supplements in their own clinic or treatment facilities. The general principles enunciated in the Act will apply in this setting, but this situation involving the health care professional is more complex and it is governed by other authorities, such as State Licensing and Registration Departments and federal kickback and antireferral statutes.

What the Act Says About...

Dietary Supplements: Includes products added to the total diet that contain at least one of the following: vitamin, mineral, herb, botanical, amino acid, another dietary substance for use to supplement the diet; or a concentrate, metabolite, constituent, extract, or combination of any ingredient described above. Products can be ingested as tablets, capsules, powder, softgel, gelcap, or liquid; must be labeled a dietary supplement; and cannot be represented for use as conventional food or sole items of a meal or diet.

Dietary supplements, including any ingredient used in them, are generally considered to be foods, but they are excluded from the definition of food additive under FDA regulations. As such, supplements cannot be regulated like food additives or drugs, which both require premarket approval regardless of the form or composition of the additive.

Unsafe Products: Under Section 4 of the DSHEA, the FDA must prove that a supplement, or an ingredient in it, presents a significant or unreasonable risk of illness or injury under conditions of use stated, or under ordinary conditions of use, if none are stated, on the label. The agency can also declare the supplement is unsafe if it contains a dietary ingredient for which there is inadequate information to provide a reasonable assurance that it does not represent risk of illness or injury. The burden of proof is with the U.S. government and, in the last case, it must inform the individual or manufacturer ten days prior to a court investigation.

The Label on the Product

Labeling — the manufacturer's claims affixed directly to the product — is a critical aspect of information transfer from manufacturer to consumer and a primary area of a manufacturer's legal responsibility. The DSHEA allows a labeling statement on a product to be made if the claim is a benefit related to a classical nutrient deficiency disease and the statement discloses the prevalence of the disease state in the United States. The label may also describe the role of a nutrient or dietary ingredient that is intended to affect the structure or function of the body, or it may characterize a documented mechanism by which a nutrient or dietary ingredient acts to maintain a bodily structure or function. Finally, the label may describe general well-being from consuming a nutrient or dietary ingredient. It would seem reasonable to have a certain degree of uniformity in dietary supplement claims, but this is unlikely to occur and is not specifically mentioned in the Act.

Problems may emerge in the area of product labeling for many manufacturers. For example, a number of dietary supplements have well-recognized effects in vitro but the conclusive demonstration of such effects in vivo may often be lacking. In addition, many alleged beneficial effects of certain dietary supplements are recorded from uncontrolled observations or are generated from epidemiologic information. These gray areas may never become distinct or even well demarcated in the near future. It is important to note that certain classes of claims for dietary supplements will likely receive intensive scrutiny by the FDA, especially those involving cancer, acquired immunodeficiency syndrome, or claims of immune modulation.

It is of utmost importance to note that labeling statements made under the DSHEA cannot make a claim to diagnose, mitigate, treat, cure, or prevent diseases. Only those specific claims linking a supplement to a disease state that have been preapproved by the FDA under the NLEA, such as soluble fiber and heart disease, may be made. The manufacturer or distributor must have substantiation that the statements used on a label are truthful and not misleading and retailers should be cautious in their presentations to consumers.

Manufacturers must notify the Secretary of Health and Human Services within thirty days after first marketing a dietary supplement. This process of notification is a passive system for the FDA, but failure to notify will be regarded as misbranding. The outcome of such a situation is difficult to anticipate, but it could result in a request by the regulatory agencies to "purge the market" of the product. One important prerequisite of all statements is that they be accompanied by a prominent display on the product or labeling documents of the following disclaimer: "This statement has not been evaluated by the Food and Drug Administration. This product is not intended to diagnose, treat, cure, or prevent any disease." This disclaimer is an attempt to distinguish dietary supplements from approved drugs that have been through the burdensome but necessary process of acceptance for marketing by the FDA.

Section 6 of the Act and relevant supporting or complementary sections are often termed the "Structure Function" provisions of the DSHEA. Any purveyor of dietary supplements that ignores these "Structure Function" provisions will not be taking full advantage of the Act as these provisions allow the truthful claims about the dietary properties of the supplement without preapproval. Manufacturers or distributors of the dietary supplement must have adequate substantiation that the labeling statements are truthful. The problem is that the degree of adequacy of the required substantiation is not defined. Manufacturers or distributors of dietary supplements are advised to collect supporting documents and produce a comprehensive database to support any labeling statement. Such a database will be essential in the event that a dispute arises with a regulatory agency.

This "Honest Label" Section of the DSHEA, Section 3, is very important. A persistent fear of the health food industry is the possibility of being issued with a misbranding charge. The ingredient labeling and nutritional information supplied to the consumer has to be accurate. Labels on dietary supplements must include: the name of each ingredient, the total weight of the ingredients, the identity of any part of the plant from which a botanical ingredient is derived, and the term "dietary supplement." Misbranding is present if the supplement claims to conform to an official standard (e.g., U.S.P.) and fails to meet the standard. If a dietary ingredient has no official standard but fails to have a composition or quality, including pharmaceutic formulation characteristics the manufacturer claims it to have, it is deemed misbranded. These regulations are designed to assist consumers in making informed decisions about the use of dietary supplements and protect them from the unscrupulous.

The DSHEA provides an amendment to earlier nutrition labeling regulations. Earlier regulations mandated that dietary supplement labels should use a conventional food nutrition facts panel, but this process has been simplified under the DSHEA. Dietary supplement labels are required to declare an amount of a substance that is required for a nutrition facts panel on conventional foods only if such substances are present in significant amounts. Doubt should be handled by disclosure.

Overseeing Labeling and Literature of Dietary Supplements

Section 12 of the DSHEA calls for the establishment of a Commission on Dietary Supplement Labels. This commission is an independent agency within the executive Branch that is charged with the responsibility to evaluate the regulation of dietary supplement label claims, labeling, and related literature. The defined need is to provide consumers with true and scientifically valid information so that they can make good judgements about self-management of their health.

The Commission on Dietary Supplement Labels will be comprised of seven members with appropriate experience and expertise. These individuals will make a final report of their activity to the President and the U.S. Congress. The Commission will have a very broad charge in order to facilitate the collection of information and coordinate hearings on matters relevant to dietary supplements. Any required rulemaking that emanates from the recommendations of the Commission will have to be completed within two years of the submission of the report of the

Commission or the final regulations on health claims for dietary supplements will be voided.

New Dietary and Grandfathered Ingredients

Section 8 of the DSHEA indicates that a dietary supplement that is first marketed after October 15, 1994, that contains an ingredient not sold prior to this date will be considered a new dietary ingredient. The DSHEA grandfathers all safe dietary supplements or ingredients that were sold prior to October 15, 1994. To be grandfathered, the product in the supplement must be unaltered from the form in which it existed, or there must be historic evidence that the product, when used as recommended, can be reasonably expected to be safe. In the event that a dietary supplement does not qualify as a "nonchemically altered food" but is not a new dietary substance because there is evidence of prior safe use or other relevant safety data, then the dietary supplement may move toward the market, providing that the Secretary of Health and Human Services is notified of these safety data seventy-five days prior to the sale of the product to a consumer. An individual or group must petition the FDA to obtain an order to permit the sale of a new dietary ingredient, but the process of the assessment of the ingredient by the FDA is likely to be stringent.

Other Issues

Under the DSHEA, it may still not be possible to claim that a dietary supplement is a good, excellent, or rich source of a particular substance unless the Secretary of Health and Human Services has issued an authorizing regulation. This area of percentage level claims covered by the Act means that the Nutrient Contents Claim Regulations are now amended to permit statements on dietary supplement labels that characterize these percentage levels, so long as the FDA has not established a reference daily intake, a daily recommended value, or any other recommendation for daily consumption of a product or nutrient. In addition, under the Act, the Proxmire Amendment (21 U.S.C. 330) is amended to include not only vitamins or minerals, but all dietary ingredients, as now defined.

Section 9 of the Act covers matters related to good manufacturing practices. The FDA may issue regulations to establish good manufacturing practices for dietary supplements that are modeled after good manufacturing practices that are currently used for foods. However, the FDA may not impose standards if no analytic methods are available, and dietary supplements that are prepared or stored under conditions that do not meet current food good manufacturing practices will be considered adulterated under the Act.

Section 11 of the Act declares that the advanced notice of proposed rule making concerning dietary supplements (58 FR 33690–33700) is declared null and void and of no effect, with a notice to be published in the Federal Register, so stating. The FDA stated its views concerning the general lack of recognition that amino acids are safe and that many herbs are really drugs. In addition, the FDA has reinforced the notion in this report that upper daily intake limits exist for vitamins and minerals, primarily to avoid toxicities.

Section 13 of the Act concerns the establishment of an Office of Dietary Supplements Research (ODSR) within the NIH. The purpose of the ODSR is to explore the role of dietary supplements to improve health and prevent disease. The Director of the ODSR is to conduct and coordinate research on dietary supplements and diseases and to act as an advisor to the Secretary of HHS, the Director of NIH, the Director of the Centers for Disease Control and Prevention, and the Commissioner of the FDA with regard to dietary supplement regulations, safety, and claims.

Conclusion

The DSHEA has far-reaching consequences for the use of dietary supplements by consumers. FDA interpretation of the Act will be a critical element in assessing the success of the DSHEA in reaching its stated goals of providing consumers with safer, properly labeled dietary supplements that are, or may be, supported with information as to their use and benefit.

To position a health food company for the future will require a team approach involving medical, scientific, and legal advice and the utilization of promotional services that are knowledgeable about the new provisions set forth in the DSHEA. On the horizon is increasing regulation, probably industry consolidation, and a rapid disappearance of those health food companies that do not have the foresight to position themselves for important regulatory issues.

Bibliography

Anderson, James W., and Breecher, Maury M. *Dr. Anderson's Antioxidant, Antiaging Health Program*. New York: Carroll and Graf Publishers, 1996.
A well-written book, well-referenced but fairly weak on discussions of herbal remedies. Likely to appeal to the supporters of integrated medicine.

Badgley, Laurence E. *Healing AIDS Naturally*. Foster City, Calif.: Healing Energy Press, 1990.
A good attempt to look at the holistic care available for AIDS. No firm recommendations, but highly recommended as a basic source of information. Somewhat outdated.

Barnett, Robert A., and Barone, Jeanine. *Ayurvedic Medicine: Ancient Roots, Modern Branches*. New York: Concorp Management, 1996.
An interesting introduction to this classic form of medicine, but the reader is somewhat misled by the disassociation of botanical remedies from the holistic nature of Ayurvedic medicine.

Bergner, Paul. *The Healing Power of Garlic: The Enlightened Person's Guide to Nature's Most Versatile Medicinal Plant*. Rocklin, Calif.: Prima Publishing, 1996.
A useful lay person's guide, with some current references.

_____. *The Healing Power of Ginseng and the Tonic Herbs: The Enlightened Person's Guide*. Rocklin, Calif.: Prima Publishing, 1996.
A useful guide for a lay person on the health benefits of ginseng.

Bland, Jeffrey. *Bioflavonoids: The Friends and Helpers of Vitamin C in Many Hard-to-Treat Ailments*. New Canaan, Conn.: Keats Publishing, 1984.
A very interesting short account of an important category of dietary supplements.

Boeser, Knut. *The Elixirs of Nostradamus: Nostradamus' Original Recipes for Elixirs, Scented Water, Beauty Potions, and Sweetmeats*. London: Bloomsbury Publishing, 1995.
Of historical interest only. For the individual who requires a classic education.

British Herbal Pharmacopoeia 1996. London: British Herbal Medicine Association, 1996.
A standard reference book. Dry but factual.

Chopra, Deepak. *Alternative Medicine: The Definitive Guide*. Fife, Wash.: Future Medicine Publishing, 1994.

A large collection of multiauthored chapters in a book that attempts to be a definitive guide to alternative medicine. Very useful as a background in alternative medicine but quite deficient in its discussion of the benefit of herbal products. Contains a surprising amount of anecdotal information and the personal biases of some authors.

Clayton, Craig, and McCullough, Virginia. *A Consumer's Guide to Alternative Health Care*. Holbrook, Mass.: Adams Publishing, 1995.
A very useful book for a lay person. Well written, informative, and grossly underestimated as a good resource.

Cook, Trevor M. *A Beginner's Introduction to Homeopathy: The Drugless Alternate Therapy That Has Healed Millions*. New Canaan, Conn.: Keats Publishing, 1987.
A useful grounding in homeopathy.

Crellin, John K., and Philpott, Jane. *Herbal Medicine Past and Present. A Reference Guide to Medicinal Plants*, vol. 2. London: Duke University Press, 1989.
Comprehensive but behind the times.

Dudley, Nigel. *Good Health on a Polluted Planet: A Handbook of Environmental Hazards and How to Avoid Them*. Hammersmith, London: Thorsons, HarperCollins Publishers, 1991.
A very useful book that may make you think twice about the conditions under which herbals or botanicals are grown.

Facklam, Margarey, and Facklam, Howard. *Healing Drugs: The History of Pharmacology*. New York: Facts on File, 1992.
A sobering, short account of drug development and natural medicine.

Fredericks, Carlton, and Bailey, Herbert. *Food Facts and Fallacies: The Intelligent Person's Guide to Nutrition and Health*. New York: Arc Books, 1971.
Very useful but dated background reading by an author who stimulates thought.

Fugh-Berman, Adriane. *Alternative Medicine: What Works: A Comprehensive Easy-to-Read Review of the Scientific Evidence, Pro and Con*. Tucson, Ariz.: Odonian Press, 1996.
A well-balanced, up-to-date book.

Fulder, Stephen. *The Book of Ginseng: And Other Chinese Herbs for Vitality*. Rochester, Vt.: Healing Arts Press, 1993.
_____ *The Ginger Book: The Ultimate Home Remedy*. Garden City Park, N.Y.: Avery Publishing Group, 1996.
Rather anecdotal in its content but one of the more complete accounts of the use of ginger.
_____ *The Handbook of Alternative and Complementary Medicine: The Most Alternative and Complete Reference Work on Complementary Therapies*. New York: Oxford University Press, 1996.

A well-written book and a good source of reference.

Grieve, M. *A Modern Herbal: The Medicinal, Culinary, Cosmetic and Economic Properties, Cultivation, and Folklore of Herbs, Grasses, Fungi, Shrubs, and Trees With All Their Modern Scientific Uses.* New York: Barnes and Noble, 1973.

The name of this book is misleading because it contains a great deal of outdated information that is largely anecdotal.

Grossinger, Richard. *Planet Medicine: Modalities.* Berkeley, Calif.: North Atlantic Books, 1996.

Entertaining reading, but quite "heavyweight." Enumerates principles without details.

————. *Planet Medicine: Origins.* Berkeley, Calif.: North Atlantic Books, 1996.

Not enough attention paid to real evidence for the benefit of herbal medicine. A little "way out."

Guide to Homeopathy. London: Brockhampton Press, 1996.

A useful book providing basic information about homeopathic options but without any hard evidence of their benefit.

Hagiwara, Yoshihide. *Green Barley Essence: The Many Health Benefits of Nature's "ideal fast food."* New Canaan, Conn.: Keats Publishing, 1985.

An exploration of the nutrient value of an increasingly popular dietary supplement.

Hedley, Christopher, and Shaw, Non. *Herbal Remedies: A Practical Beginner's Guide to Making Effective Remedies in the Kitchen.* Bristol, England: Parragon Books Service, 1996.

A nice picture book containing a lot of outdated recommendations. Useful as a very basic introduction.

Heinerman, John. *Aloe Vera, Jojoba and Yucca: The Amazing Health Benefits They Can Give You.* New Canaan, Conn.: Keats Publishing, 1982.

A somewhat anecdotal account of some potentially useful botanicals.

Hoffer, Abram, and Walker, Morton. *Smart Nutrients: A Guide to Nutrients That Can Prevent and Reverse Senility.* Garden City Park, N.Y.: Avery Publishing Group, 1994.

An interesting book with good basics and lateral thinking.

Holt, Stephen. *Soya for Health: The Definitive Medical Guide.* Larchmont, N.Y.: Mary Ann Liebert, 1996.

A book written for a health care giver, it is tough reading for a lay person. Written in a highly referenced format to attempt to provide a definitive medical guide on soybeans and health.

Jacobs, Jennifer. *The Encyclopedia of Alternative Medicine.* Boston: Journey Editions, Charles E. Tuttle Co., 1996.

An easy read to gain an overall background, but somewhat deficient in facts.

Kaptchuk, Ted J. *The Web That Has No Weaver: Understanding Chinese Medicine.*

Chicago: Congdon and Weed, 1983.

Tough reading, but essential if an individual wants to apply traditional Chinese medical herbal products. The empiric basis of the use of Chinese herbs becomes apparent by studying the principles of Chinese medicine.

Kaptchuk, Ted J. and Croucher, Michael. *The Healing Arts: A Journey Through the Faces of Medicine.* London: British Broadcasting Corp., 1986.

A great read but little factual information.

Keys, John D. *Chinese Herbs: Their Botany, Chemistry, and Pharmacodynamics.* Bunkyo-ku, Japan: Charles E. Tuttle Co., 1976.

A useful book about some of the main types of herbs used in Chinese medicine. The book is deficient in medical references but a useful overall source of information.

Kloss, Jethro. *Back to Eden: The Classic Guide to Herbal Medicine, Natural Foods, and Home Remedies.* Loma Linda, Calif.: Back to Eden Books, 1994.

A classic book that is so outdated in many sections that it could be construed as misleading.

Koch, Heinrich P., and Lawson, Larry D. *Garlic: The Science and Therapeutic Application of Allium sativum L. and Related Species.* Baltimore, Maryland: Williams and Wilkins, 1996.

The definitive guide to garlic and related herbs, highly recommended.

Lalitha, Thomas. *Ten Essential Herbs: Everyone's Handbook to Health.* Prescott, Ariz.: Hohm Press, 1992.

Very anecdotal but contains some practical hints.

Lee, William H., and Rosenbaum, Michael. *Chlorella: The Sun-Powered Supernutrient and Its Beneficial Properties.* New Canaan, Conn.: Keats Publishing, 1987.

A short guide to the potential health benefit of chlorella, peppered with anecdotal information.

Levine, Stephen A., and Kidd, Parris M. *Antioxidant Adaptation: Its Role in Free Radical Pathology.* San Leandro, Calif.: Allergy Research Group, 1986.

An excellent, serious book that is hard reading for anyone with less than a "technical" interest in antioxidants. An example of serious scientific pursuit to be highly commended in the dietary supplement industry.

Lu, Henry C. *Chinese Herbal Cures.* New York: Sterling Publishing Co., 1991.

Hard to read, impossible to decipher; contains little clear guidance on how to use Chinese medicine.

Lucas, Richard. *Secrets of the Chinese Herbalists.* West Nyack, N.Y.: Parker Publishing Company, 1977.

A nice synopsis for a lay reader but overreaching in its conclusions.

Lust, John. *The Herb Book: The Most Complete Catalog of Nature's "Miracle Plants" Ever Published.* New York: Bantam Books, 1974.

Of major interest from the botanical perspective but uncertain on the health application of herbs.

Majeed, Muhammed; Badmaev, Vladimir; and Frank, Murray. *Turmeric and the Healing Curcuminoids: Their Amazing Antioxidant Properties and Protective Powers.* New Canaan, Conn.: Keats Publishing, 1996.
A useful account of the health benefit of tumeric.

Marsh, Edward E. *How to Be Healthy With Natural Foods.* New York: Gramercy Publishing Company, 1963.
A very understandable book that is deficient in facts. Very "dated" concepts.

Mayell, Mark. *Off-the-Shelf Natural Health: How to Use Herbs and Nutrients to Stay Well.* London: Boxtree Limited, 1995.
An excellent book, well written, appropriately conservative in its claims and quite understandable to a lay person.

Moore, Natasha. *Traditional Natural Skin Care: A Starter's Guide to Making Your Own Beauty Preparations, Using Pure, Fresh and Natural Ingredients.* Bristol, England: Parragon Book Service, 1996.
A very nice synopsis of some "quaint" topical remedies to improve skin beauty and health.

Mowrey, Daniel B. *Echinacea: How an Amazing Herb Supports and Stimulates Your System.* New Canaan, Conn.: Keats Publishing, 1995.
An excellent guide to this very useful herb, well written and readable.

_____. *Herbal Tonic Therapies: Remedies From Nature's Own Pharmacy to Strengthen and Support Each Vital Body System.* New Canaan, Conn.: Keats Publishing, 1993.
A well-written book with adequate references but some overoptimistic conclusions about the benefit of herbs in some disease states. Highly recommended.

_____. *Next Generation Herbal Medicine: Guaranteed Potency Herbs.* New Canaan, Conn.: Keats Publishing, 1990.
A useful reference book for a health care giver.

_____. *The Scientific Validation of Herbal Medicine: How to Remedy and Prevent Disease With Herbs, Vitamins, Minerals and Other Nutrients.* New Canaan, Conn.: Keats Publishing, 1986.
A good attempt to summarize some of the scientific evidence to support the health benefits of herbs.

Murray, Michael T. *The Healing Power of Herbs: The Enlightened Person's Guide to the Wonders of Medicinal Plants.* Rocklin, Calif.: Prima Publishing, 1995.
An excellent book that is well written and well referenced, highly recommended.

Naturopathic Handbook of Herbal Formulas: A Practical and Concise Herb User's Guide. Ayer, Mass.: Herbal Research Publications, 1995.
Didactic, laconic, difficult to read, and poorly referenced. Claims to

incorporate holistic approaches but provides little credible scientific evidence to support the proposed concoctions.

Nuzzi, Debra. *Pocket Herbal Reference Guide*. Freedom, Calif.: Crossing Press, 1992. A list of questionable applications of many herbs.

Passwater, Richard A. *A Beginner's Introduction to Vitamins: The Fundamental Necessities for Growth and Maintenance of Life*. New Canaan, Conn.: Keats Publishing, 1983.
An essential basis for the uninformed lay reader.

————. and Kandaswami, Chithan. *Super "Protector" Nutrient*. New Canaan, Conn.: Keats Publishing, 1994.
A short book loaded with facts but deficient in support for its conclusions in many areas.

Pizzorno, Joseph. *Total Wellness: Improve Your Health by Understanding the Body's Healing Systems*. Rocklin, Calif.: Prima Publishing, 1996.
An excellent approach to developing treatment programs that involve remedies of natural origin. Well referenced and well balanced. This book is likely to be rejected by a conventional physician, but it contains a great deal of common sense and lateral thought.

Puotinen, C.J. *Herbal Teas: Brewing and Blending the Delicious, Restorative Drinks That Can Heal, Calm or Energize Your Body*. New Canaan, Conn.: Keats Publishing, 1996.
A very useful guide for a lot of people.

Robbins, Christopher. *Herbalism: An Introductory Guide*. Hammersmith, London: Diamond Books, 1995.
Good basic reading.

Rogers, Sherry A. *Chemical Sensitivity: Environmental Diseases and Pollutants — How They Hurt Us, How to Deal With Them*. New Canaan, Conn.: Keats Publishing, 1995.
An interesting booklet that draws everyone's attention to diseases determined by environmental influences, especially pollutants.

Rosenberg, Harold. *Nutrition and Stress: Only Total Health Awareness Can Help Us Survive*. New Canaan, Conn.: Keats Publishing, 1983.
A short, useful account of holistic health approaches.

Schachter, Michael B. *The Natural Way to a Healthy Prostate: Preventing Prostate Problems With Nutritional and Herbal Treatments*. New Canaan, Conn.: Keats Publishing, 1995.
An excellent synopsis of complementary medical approaches to the treatment of prostatic disease.

Schauss, Alexander. *The Health Benefits of Cat's Claw: Its Role in Treating Cancer, Arthritis, Prostate Problems, Asthma and Many Other Chronic Conditions*. New Canaan, Conn.: Keats Publishing, 1996.

An attempt to summarize evidence for a medical benefit of cats claw in the presence of little hard scientific fact.

Sears, Barry, and Lawren, William. *Enter the Zone: A Dietary Road Map to: Lose Weight Permanently, Reset Your Genetic Code, Prevent Disease, Achieve Maximum Physical Performance, Enhance Mental Productivity.* New York: Regan Books, HarperCollins Publishers, 1995.

An interesting book with many innovative concepts.

Seibold, Ronald L. *Cereal Grasses: The Concentrated Health-Giving Power of Green Barley, Wheat and Other Grains at Their Nutrient Peak.* New Canaan, Conn.: Keats Publishing, 1996.

An interesting account of the variety of nutrients in cereal grasses.

Simopoulos, Artemis P.; Herbert, Victor; and Jacobson, Beverley. *The Healing Diet: How to Reduce Your Risks and Live a Longer and Healthier Life If You Have a Family History of Cancer, Heart Disease, Hypertension, Diabetes, Alcoholism, Obesity, Food Allergies.* New York: Macmillan, 1995.

Very informative, well-balanced, with good practical advice. Very useful in understanding how important it is to look at facts when considering nutritional interventions.

Smyth, Angela. *The Complete Encyclopaedia of Natural Health.* London:Thorsons, HarperCollins Publishers, 1997.

A useful overview of natural options for a variety of disease states.

Stanway, Andrew. *Alternative Medicine: A Guide to Natural Therapies.* London: Chancellor Press, 1986.

An excellent overview of complementary medicine. Highly recommended with well-balanced conclusions.

Taylor, Christopher E. *Nutritional Abnormalities in Infectious Diseases: Effects on Tuberculosis and AIDS.* Binghamton, N.Y.: Haworth Medical Press, 1997.

An overlooked area that explains the importance of nutrition in infectious disease.

Treacher, Sylvia. *Practical Homeopathy: A Beginner's Guide to Natural Remedies for Use in the Home.* Bristol, England: Parragon Book Service, 1996.

This book attempts to turn individuals into homeopathic "self-medicators." Homeopathy is best applied by a homeopathic physician or healer.

Tyler, V.E. *The Honest Herbal: A Sensible Guide to the Use of Herbs and Related Remedies.* 3rd ed. Binghamton, N.Y.: Pharmaceutical Products Press, Haworth Press, 1993.

One of the best books available on commonly used herbal remedies. The author is unwilling to give any anecdotal information or the benefit of any doubt when reaching a conclusion. Probably requires further updating, especially in relationship to several herbal remedies that have been the focus of recent research. The author comes across with a degree of skepticism that is somewhat off-putting for practitioners of complementary medicine. The book is well referenced and highly recommended.

Ullman, Dana. *Discovering Homeopathy: Your Introduction to the Science and Art of Homeopathic Medicine.* Berkeley, Calif.: North Atlantic Books, 1991.

An interesting dialogue that is well referenced on classic homeopathic approaches.

_____. *The Consumer's Guide to Homeopathy: The Definitive Resource for Understanding Homeopathic Medicine and Making It Work for You.* New York: G. P. Putman's Sons, 1995.

A very useful book. Like many homeopathic books, it contains many anecdotes, but there is a serious attempt to provide references on many homeopathic remedies.

Vries, Jan de. *Melissa Extract: The Natural Herbal Remedy for Herpes: Safe Treatment for One of the Most Widespread and Insidious Diseases.* New Canaan, Conn.: Keats Publishing, 1996.

An anecdotal account of a promising herbal approach to a "rotten" disease.

Wardlaw, Gordon M., and Insel, Paul M. *Perspectives in Nutrition.* St. Louis: Mosby-Year Book, 1993.

A comprehensive book providing basic grounding on sound nutritional facts.

Werbach, Melvyn R. *Nutritional Influences on Illness: A Sourcebook of Clinical Research.* 2nd ed. Tarzana, Calif.: Third Line Press, 1993.

An excellent resource.

Werbach, Melvin R., and Murray, Michael T. *Botanical Influences on Illness: A Sourcebook of Clinical Research.* Tarzana, Calif.: Third Line Press, 1994.

An excellent book, well referenced but requiring updating for health care givers. One of the most useful books in alternative medicine.

Woodward, Marcus. *Gerard's Herbal.* London: Senate, Studio Editions, 1994.

Only of use to those interested in history but a necessary part of the classic education of a serious herbalist.

Wunderlich, Ray C. *Natural Alternatives to Antibiotics: The Safe Remedies That Work With Your Body to Fight Illness.* New Canaan, Conn.: Keats Publishing, 1995.

An interesting approach that requires more substantiation.

Index

About the Authors

Stephen Holt, M.D., MRCP (UK), FRCP (C), FACP, FACG, FACN, is the president and chief executive officer of BioTherapies, Inc. The New Jersey corporation is engaged in the research and development of remedies of natural origin.

Dr. Holt has formulated more than twenty natural remedies that are numbered among the bestselling products in the worldwide dietary supplement industry. The author of several hundred scientific communications and several books on conventional and natural medicine, he has contributed to the research and development of several prescription medications. Recipient of many awards for the postgraduate teaching of medicine, he is a frequent guest lecturer at university and scientific meetings throughout the world. He has held several appointments in academic medicine at universities in England, Canada, the United States, and China and has practiced medicine for twenty-five years. Dr. Holt's current collaborative medical research involves academic colleagues in China, Taiwan, Costa Rica, and Korea.

Linda Comac received both her B.A. and M.A. in English from the City University of New York. A teacher of English, journalism, and creative writing at both the high school and college levels for more than two decades, she is the author of numerous newspaper and magazine articles and two books. Ms. Comac's interest in medicine grew around the dinner tables of her childhood, where her father — a pharmacist — and her uncle — a physician — often discussed the issues of the times. The subsequent untimely deaths of her father, her aunt, and two lifelong friends to heart failure, leukemia, lupus, and AIDS, respectively, led her to question allopathic medicine. When not writing or teaching, she is busy raising two sons.